Phytochemicals for
Diabetic Complications

Phytochemicals for Diabetic Complications

Prof. (Dr). Ciddi Veeresham
Principal
Faculty of Pharmacy
Sri Ramachandra Institute of
Higher Education and Research
(Deemed to be University)
Porur, Chennai-600 116
Tamil Nadu

Dr. Ajmera Rama Rao
Post-Doctoral Fellow
University College of Pharmaceutical Sciences
Kakatiya University
Warangal-506001 (TS)

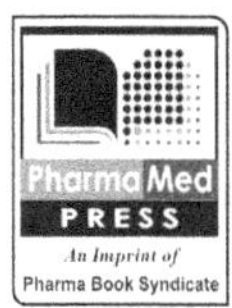

PharmaMed Press

An imprint of Pharma Book Syndicate
A unit of BSP Books Pvt. Ltd.
4-4-309/316, Giriraj Lane,
Sultan Bazar, Hyderabad - 500 095.

Phytochemicals for Diabetic Complications
by Prof. (Dr). Ciddi Veeresham and Dr. Ajmera Rama Rao

Published by :

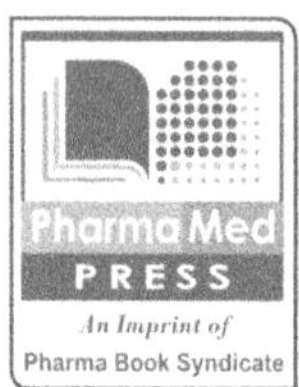

PharmaMed Press
An imprint of Pharma Book Syndicate
A unit of BSP Books Pvt. Ltd.
4-4-309/316, Giriraj Lane, Sultan Bazar, Hyderabad - 500 095.
Phone: 040-23445688, 23445600; Fax: 91+40-23445611
e-mail: info@pharmamedpress.com
www.pharmamedpress.com/pharmamedpress.net

ISBN : 978-93-89974-17-1

Preface

Diabetes Mellitus (DM) is a chronic disorder of impaired metabolism of carbohydrates, fats and proteins characterized by hyperglycemia resulting from decreased utilization of carbohydrate and excessive glycogenolysis from amino acids and fatty acids. People with DM are at higher risk of developing serious complications such as diabetic nephropathy, diabetic retinopathy, and peripheral neuropathy including heart attack, blindness and Kidney failure. Four molecular mechanisms are being extensively studied for their role in causing diabetic complications; increase in the flux of glucose through polyol pathway, increased intracellular formation of advanced glycation end-products (AGES), activation of protein kinase C (PKC) and in created flux through the hexosamine pathway; Aldose reductase enzyme is involved in the polyol pathway will be converted glucose to sorbitol and further involved in the development of diabetic complication.

Even though a large variety of compounds have been synthesized with potent *in-vitro* aldose reductase inhibitory activity (ARI), very few compounds are clinically available because of undesirable side effects and poor Pharmacokinetics. The failure of these compounds has increased the need for search of newer molecules from natural sources. To date number as plant extracts and their phyto constituents have reported to have aldose reductase activity to treat the diabetic complications.

The book starts with a chapter as Aldose reductase inhibitors on phyto constituents, *in-vitro* screening methods for Rat kidney Aldose reductase inhibitory activity, Aldose reductase enzyme from Bovine Eyes, Human Recombinant Aldose reductase inhibitory activity including *in-vivo* methods. It also discussed about the phytochemicals screened do for AR inhibitory activity. The second chapter deals with plant extracts studied for AR inhibitory activity. Chapter 3 describes about plants and phytochemicals used as Anti-glycation Agents and used in the management of diabetic complication. Chapter 4 has been given about the pants used in the management of diabetic complications. Last chapter 5 has been specifically the herbal medicine used in the diabetic foot complications.

Each chapter is profusely illustrated with figures tables and chemical structures and attempts to convey the practical as well as theoretical aspects. It should, therefore, find application for people working area of Diabetes complications.

We have made a humble attempt to present the subject in lucid manner and have taken all possible care to avoid mistaken. One of the authors expresses his sincere gratitude to Sri. V.R. Venkataachalam, Honourable Chancellor of Sri Ramachandra Institute of Higher Education and Research (SRIHER), Chennai for his kind patronage of this endeavour of mine. Heartfelt thanks are owed to Sri R.V. Sengutuvan, Pro-chancellor and Dr. P.V. Vijayaraghavan, Vice-Chancellor Sri Ramachandra Institute of Higher education and research (SRIHER), Chennai for his cheerful patronage and Friendship.

Prof. (Dr). Ciddi Veeresham

Dr. Ajmera Rama Rao

Contents

CHAPTER 1

Aldose Reductase Inhibitors Phyto Constituents

CHAPTER 2

Aldose Reductase Inhibitors from Plant Extracts

Chapter 1

Aldose Reductase Inhibitors Phyto Constituents

1.1 Introduction

India has become the capital of diabetic. According to a report by IDF (international diabetes federation 2015), 1 in 7 births is affected by gestational diabetes,1 in 11 adults have diabetes (415 million), by 2040, 1 adult in 10 (642 million) will have diabetes, Every 6 seconds a person dies from diabetes (5.0 million deaths).

People with diabetes are at higher risk of developing a number of disabling and life-threatening health problems than people without diabetes. Consistently high blood glucose levels can lead to serious diseases affecting the heart and blood vessels, eyes, kidneys and nerves. People with diabetes are also at increased risk of developing infections. In almost all high-income countries, diabetes is a leading cause of cardiovascular disease, blindness, kidney failure and lower-limb amputation (IDF 2015).

Therefore, there is a growing interest in search of drugs that alleviate the various symptoms of diabetic complications. Several studies have suggested that hyperglycaemia may have important role in the pathogenesis of diabetic complications by several mechanisms. Of these, increased aldose reductase (AR) related polyol pathway flux is one important mechanism (Brownlee, 2001). AR is an NADPH-dependent oxidoreductase and one of the important enzymes in the polyol pathway (Figure 1.1) that catalyses the reduction of various sugars to sugar alcohols, such as glucose to sorbitol. Sorbitol is then catalyzed to fructose by sorbitol dehydrogenase, an NADPH-dependent enzyme. Under normal conditions, the affinities of cell based AR for glucose are low, however, in diabetic conditions; an increase in the rate of the AR related polyol pathway augments intracellular concentrations of sorbitol and its metabolite fructose. As shown in Figure 1, accumulation of sorbitol in the cells due to its poor penetration across membranes and inefficient metabolism results in the development of diabetic complications (Kador *et al.*, 1980).

1

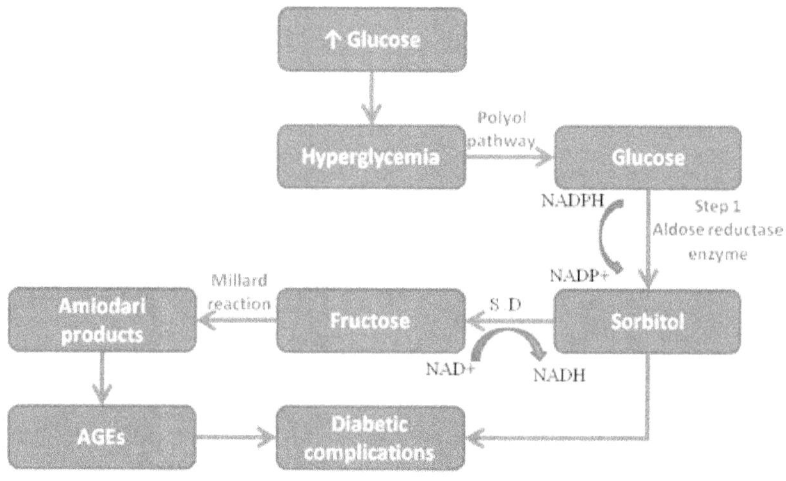

Figure 1.1 Schematic diagram presenting the process for the development of complications of Diabetes mellitus (Chethan *et al.*, 2008). S.D: sorbitol dehydrogenase.

The polyol pathway plays an important role in the development of degenerative complications of diabetes, such as neuropathy, nephropathy, retinopathy, cataract and cardiovascular diseases (Wirasathien et *al.*, 2007). The other mechanisms like increased advanced glycation end-product (AGE) formation, activation of protein kinase C (PKC) isoforms and increased hexosamine pathway flux also contribute to diabetic complications. All these mechanisms emphasize hyperglycaemia-induced overproduction of superoxides involving the mitochondrial electron-transport chain (Brownlee., 2001).

In the Western world the incidence of diabetes mellitus is increasing at an almost epidemic rate. Because of this high incidence and the associated morbidity and mortality, it has become a major health hazard. The diabetes control and complications trial (DCCT) undertaken in the USA in 1993; the United Kingdom prospective diabetes study (UKPDS) conducted in 1998, and a Japanese trial have all demonstrated that strict and sustained control of glucose excursions through interventions, including intensive insulin therapy, reduces the risk of developing these complications in diabetics, thereby showing the association between hyperglycaemia and the development of long-term diabetic complications (Ohkubo *et al.,* 1995). However, close control is difficult to maintain, and considerable efforts have been made to find novel and effective antidiabetic agents that act by mechanisms independent of controlling blood glucose. AR inhibitors (ARIs) offer the possibility of preventing or arresting the progression of these long-term diabetic complications, despite the high blood glucose levels and hence with no risk of hypoglycaemia, since they have no effect on blood glucose (Costantino *et al.*, 1999). The present book gives an insight into the screening methods that are commonly employed for AR inhibitory activity and also summarizes phytochemicals and extracts which have been reported to possess AR inhibitory activity.

Screening Methods for AR Inhibitory Activity

AR inhibitory activity is screened by both *in vitro* and *in vivo* methods. *In vitro* assays for AR enzyme are further classified into different models based on source of enzyme.

In vitro Methods

Rat lens AR (RLAR) inhibitory activity. Male albino rats of wister strain weighing 250-280 g are used for isolation of crude AR. Rat lens homogenate is prepared according to the modified method of Hayman *et al.* (1965) whereby the lenses are homogenized in sodium phosphate buffer (pH 6.2) and the supernatant obtained by centrifugation of the homogenate at 10000 rpm at 4 °C for 20 min is frozen until use. Crude AR, with activity of 6.5 U/mg, is used for the evaluation of enzyme inhibition. Reaction solution consisting of 600 μL of 100 mM of sodium phosphate buffer (pH 6.2), 100 μL of AR homogenate, 100 μL of 0.15 μM NADPH, 9 μL of the sample dissolved in 10% DMSO and 90 μL of 50 mM of DL-glyceraldehyde as the substrate. The AR activity is determined by measuring the decrease in NADPH absorption at 340 nm over 4 min period on UV/Visble spectrophotometer.

Rat Kidney AR (RKAR) Inhibitory Activity

In this method male albino rats of wister strain weighing 250-280 g are used for isolation of crude AR. Rat kidney homogenate is prepared according to the modified method outlined by Cerelli *et al.* (1986). The kidneys are first homogenized in sodium phosphate buffer (pH 6.2) and the supernatant obtained by centrifugation of the homogenate at 4000 rpm at 4 °C for 30 min is then frozen until use. Crude AR, with activity of 6.5 U/mg, is used for the evaluation of enzyme inhibition. Reaction solution is made to contain 1.0 mL of 100 mM sodium phosphate buffer (pH 6.2), 100 μL of AR homogenate, 100 μL of 0.15 μM NADPH, 100 μL of the sample (different concentrations prepared in DMSO) and100 μL of 100 mM of DL-glyceraldehyde as a substrate. AR activity is determined by measuring the decrease in NADPH absorption at 340 nm over 1 min period. Quercetin, a well-known ARI, is generally used as a reference standard.

AR Enzyme from Cataracted Human Eye Lens

Cataracted human eye lenses are washed with saline and their fresh weights are recorded. The lenses are pooled and homogenized in (1:2 w/v) sodium phosphate buffer (0.135 M, pH 7.0) containing 0.5 mM phenylmethyl sulfonyl fluoride (PMSF) and 10 mM β-mercaptoethanol and centrifuged at 8000g for 30 min at 4 °C. The supernatant is used for determination of AR activity (Chethan *et al.*, 2008).

AR Enzyme from Bovine Eyes

In this method the AR enzyme is obtained from bovine eyes lenses. The lenses are removed by lateral incision of the eye and homoginized in 135 mM phosphate buffer containing 10 mM β-mercaptoethanol. The homogenate is centrifuged at 10000g for 15 min and the supernatant fluid used for determination of AR activity (Guzman *et al.*, 2005).

Human Recombinant AR (HRAR) Inhibitory Activity

Inhibition of HRAR is determined according to the method described by Nishimura *et al.* (1991). The reaction mixture is prepared by mixing 100 µL 0.15 mM NADPH, 100 µL of 10 mM DL-glyceraldehyde (as a substrate), 5 µL HRAR and various concentrations of the sample with 100 mM sodium phosphate buffer (pH 6.2) to adjust the total volume to 1 mL. AR activity is determined by measuring the decrease in NADPH absorption at 340 nm over a period of 1 min.

PL (porcine lens) AR Inhibitory Activity

Lenses were removed from porcine eyes and homoginized in 3 vol of 135 mM phosphate buffer containing 10 mM β-mercaptoethanol. The homogenate is centrifuged at 10000g for 15 min and the supernatant fluid used for determination of AR activity (Haraguchi *et al.*, 1996).

In vivo Methods

Determination of lens galactitol levels by GLC. Lens galactitol level is determined according to the method of Kato *et al.* (2006). After 21 days of feeding galactose, rats are sacrificed by CO_2 asphyxiation and the eyeballs surgically excised. The lenses are carefully dissected under sterile conditions, the lens material weighed and homogenized in 20% ice cold acetonitrile (1 mL). The sample and methyl α-D-mannopyranoside (0.1 µM) used as internal standard are mixed, centrifuged to eliminate proteins and the resulting supernatant lyophilized. Sugar alcohols are trimethysilylated using tri-sil reagent. After addition of 1 mL of the silylating reagent, the tube is placed in an incubating oven at 60 °C for 30 min. Analysis is performed by GLC.

Estimation of Galactitol Levels in Galactosomic Rat Lens by RP-HPLC

Lyophilized samples of five groups of galactosomic rat were derivatized by adding 250µL of pyridine and 500µL of phenylisocynate and the reaction carried out for 1hr at 55^0C on water bath with occasionally shaking. Derivatized samples are analyzed by reverse-phase C 18 column with the ultraviolet detector at 240 nm. HPLC run by using mobile phase consisting of acetonitrile and 0.01M dipotassium hydrogen phosphate buffer (60:40). Flow rate was adjusted to 2 mL/min and the injection volume was 20 µL. A standard graph was plotted by analyzing solutions of different concentrations of galactitol using glucose as internal standard.

Phytochemicals with AR Inhibitory Activity

Although several synthetic ARIs such as tolrestat, epalrestat and sorbinil exhibit potent effects, either their use was limited, or they have been withdrawn from clinical trials because of relatively low efficacy, poor pharmacokinetics and unsatisfactory safety (Kawannishi *et al.*, 2003; Manzanaro *et al.*, 2006; Peyrou *et al.,* 2006). At present, only eplarestat, which reached the Japanese market in 1992, is still available in Japan. Thus, there is still an urgent need for development of improved ARIs (Angel de la Fuente and Manzanaro, (2003)).

There is growing interest in the benefits of dietary supplements such as naturceuticals and traditional herbal medicines as pharmaceuticals that lack toxicity and other harmful side effects. A vast literature survey showed that cataract progression could be slowed or prevented by inhibition of AR enzyme using natural resources (Crabbe *et al.*, 1998; Fuente *et al.*, 2003).

Many structurally diverse phytochemicals and extracts have been reported as potent ARIs *in vitro*. Currently known ARIs can be classified into four main groups based on their structures: acetic acid derivatives e.g. tolrestat and epalrestat, cyclic imides e.g. sorbini, phenolic derivatives e.g. quercetin, and phenylsulfonyl nitromethane derivatives e.g. ZD 5522.

Plant derived compounds having significant AR inhibitory activity can be classified into specific chemical groups such as flavonoids, tannins, phenolics, alkaloids, terpenoids, coumarins and miscellaneous compounds. The structures of these phytochemicals are shown in Figures 2-7.

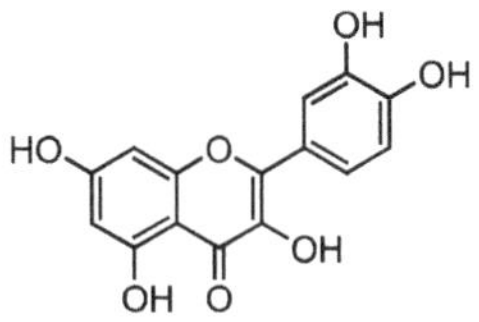

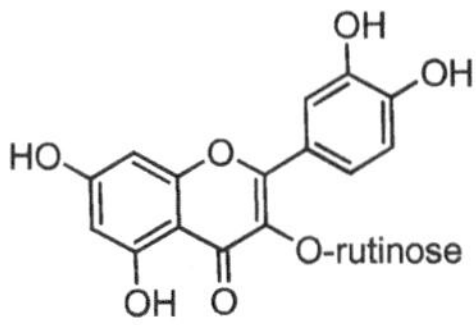

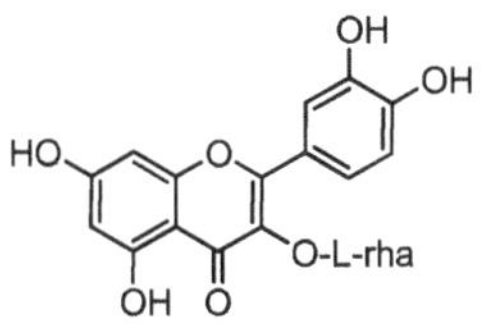

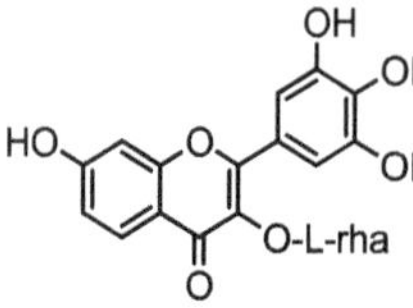

(4)

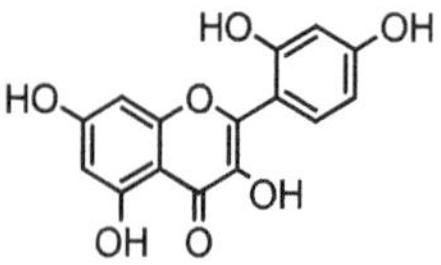

(5)

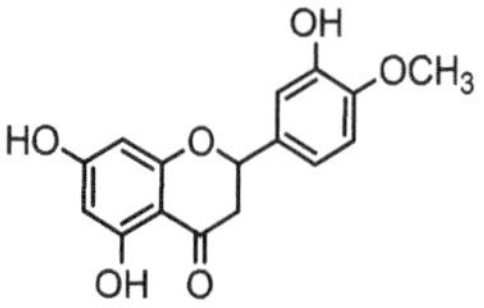

(6)

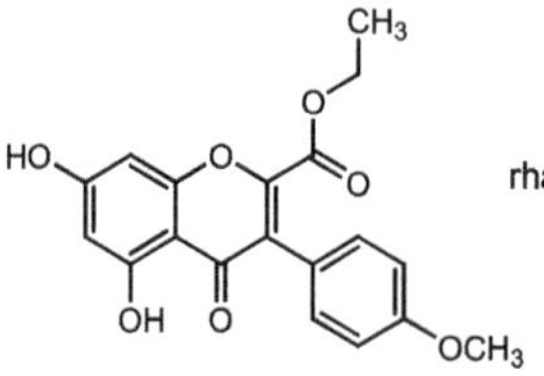

(7)

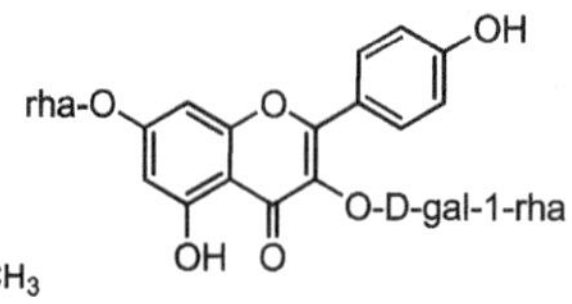

(8)

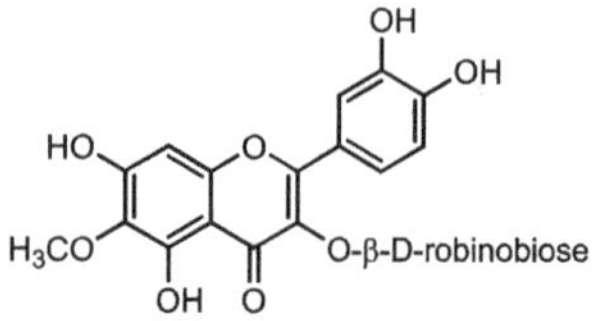

(9)

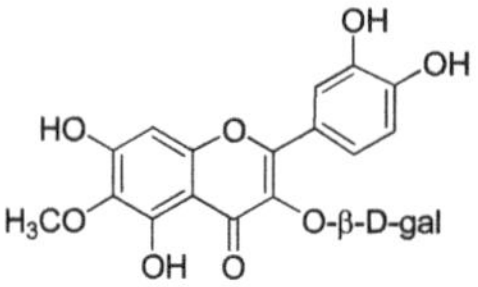

(10)

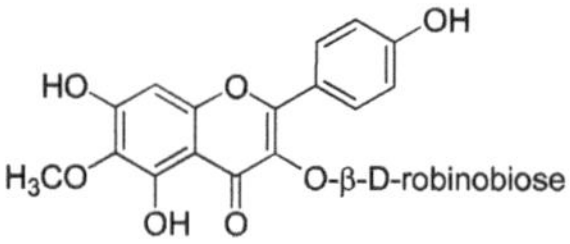

(11)

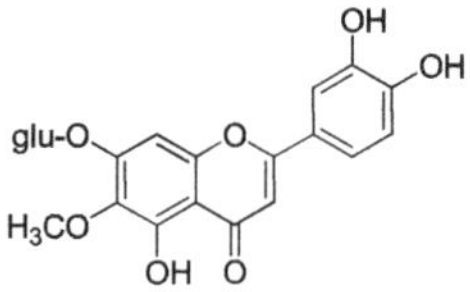

(12)

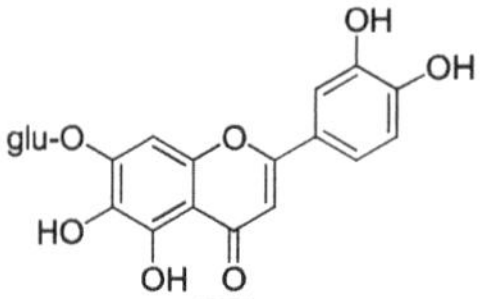

(13)

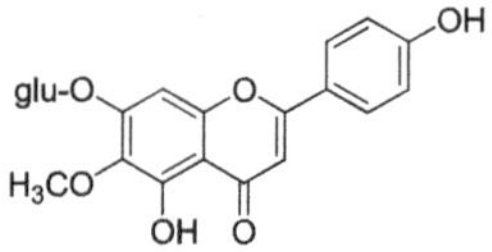

(14)

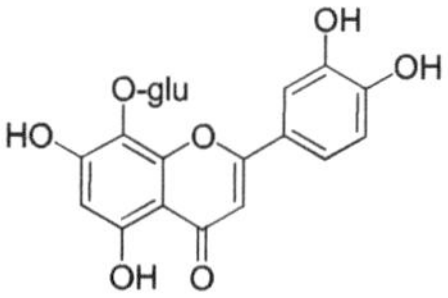

(15)

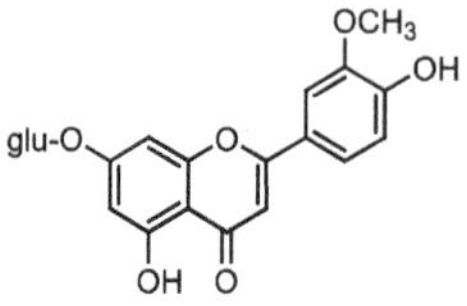

(16)

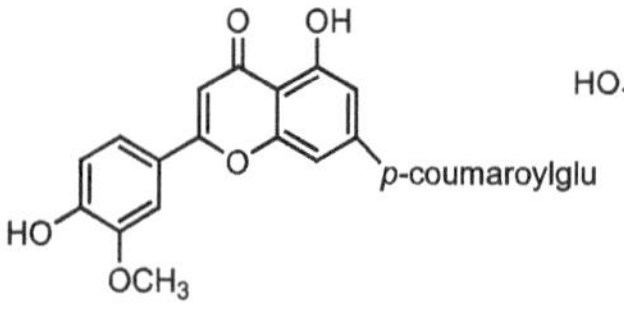

(17)

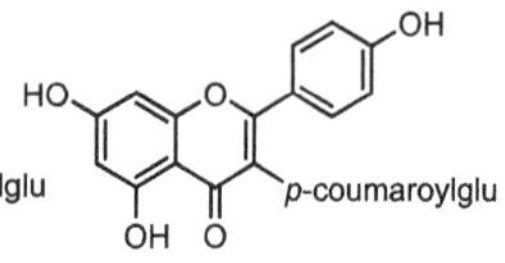

(18)

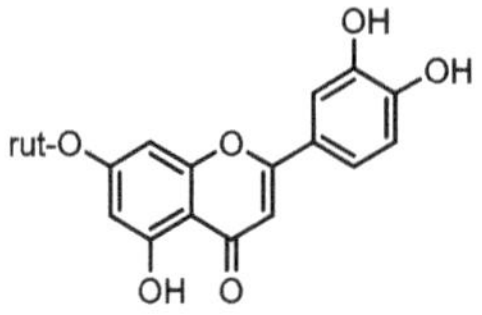

(19)

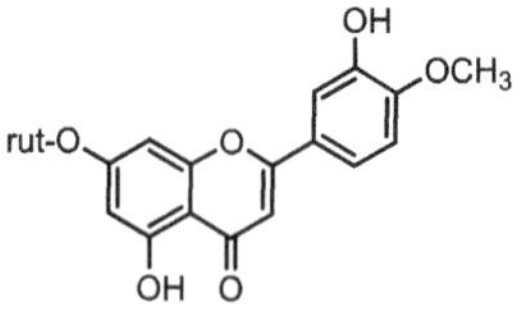

(20)

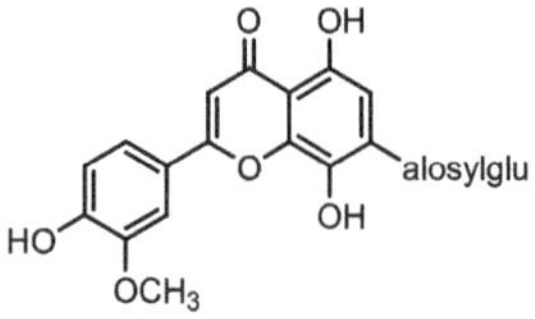

(21)

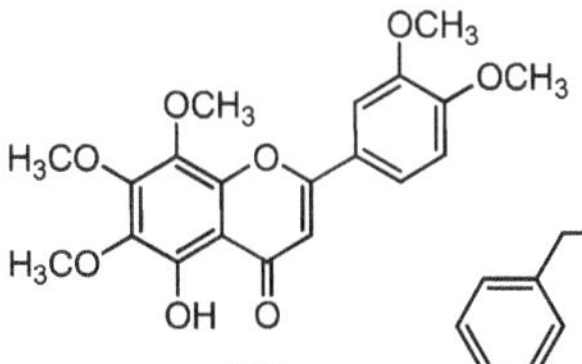

(25)

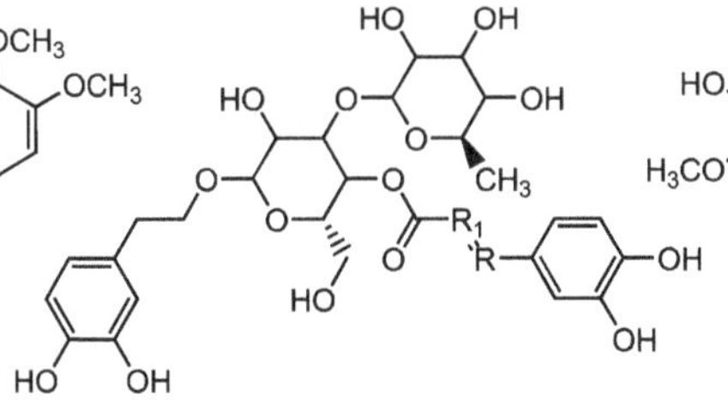

R-R1 =single bond   acteoside **(26)**
R-R1 = double bond   dehydroacteoside **(27)**

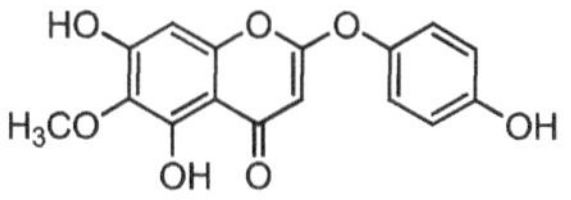

(28)

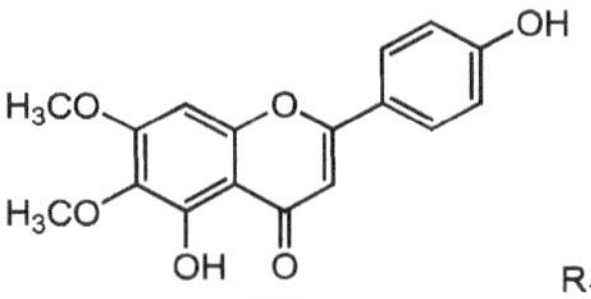

(29)

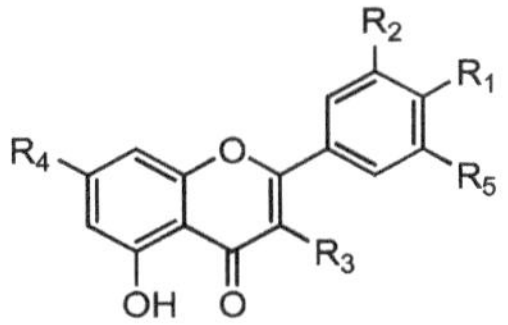

R$_1$	R$_2$	R$_3$	R$_4$	R$_5$	
OH	OH	OSO$_3$K	OH	H	**(30)**
OH	OCH$_3$	OH	OH	H	**(31)**
OH	OCH$_3$	OSO$_3$K	OH	H	**(32)**
OH	OCH$_3$	OSO$_3$K	OSO$_3$K	H	**(33)**
OH	OCH$_3$	OH	OCH$_3$	H	**(34)**
OH	OCH$_3$	OSO$_3$K	OCH$_3$	H	**(35)**
OH	OH	O-glu	OH	H	**(36)**
OCH$_3$	H	O-glu	OSO$_3$K	OH	**(37)**

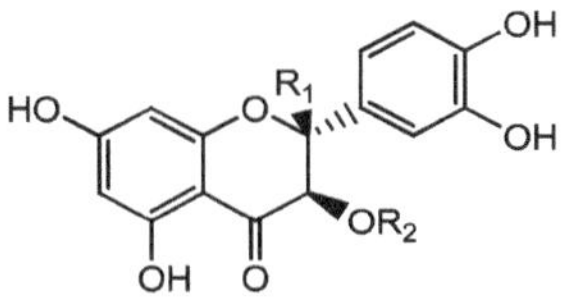

R$_1$=H R$_2$=H   **(38)**
R$_1$=H R$_2$= rha **(39)**

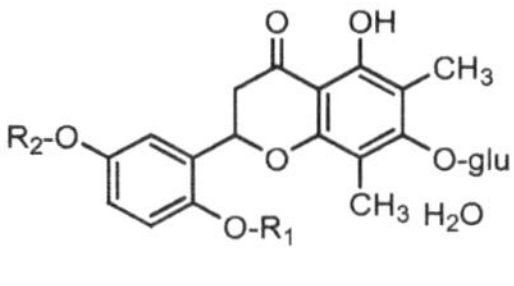

R$_1$ = R$_2$ = H   **(40)**
R$_1$ = H R$_2$ = CH$_3$ **(41)**

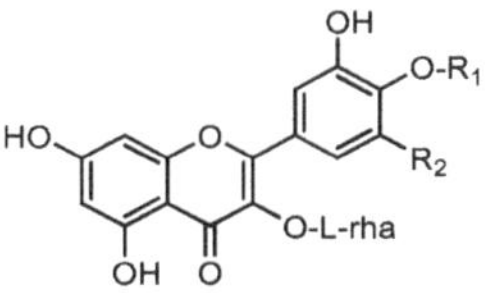

R$_1$ = H   R$_2$ = OH **(42)**
R$_1$ = CH3 R$_2$ = OH **(43)**

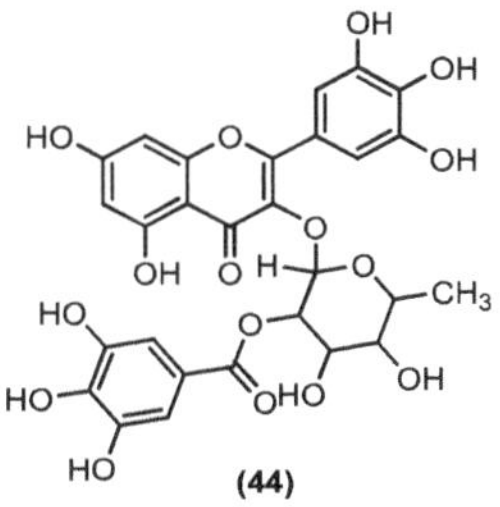

(44)

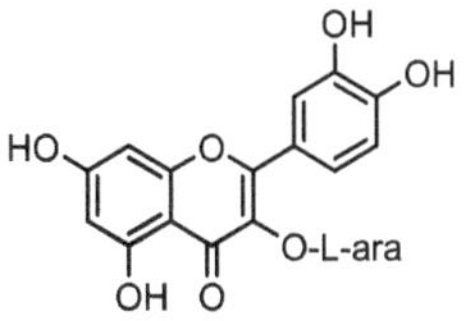

(45)

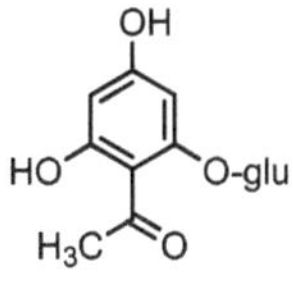

(46)

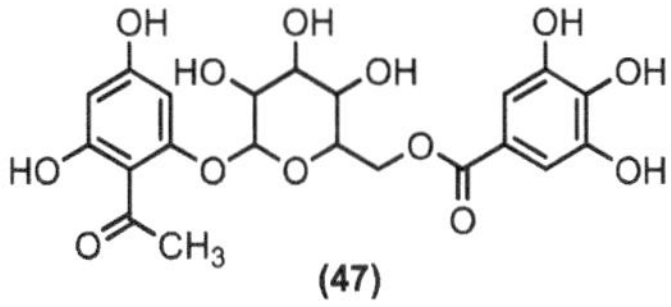

(47)

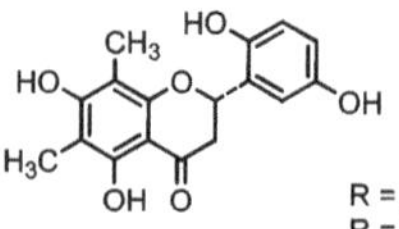

(48)

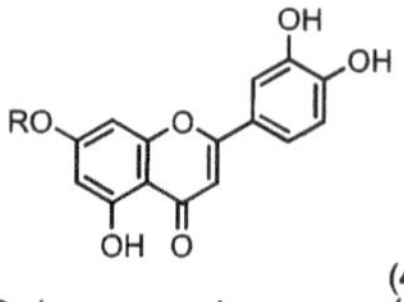

R = H (49)
R = β-D-glucopyranosyl (50)
R = β-D-glucopyranosiduronic acid (51)

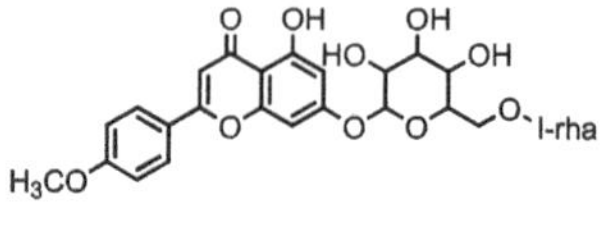

(52)

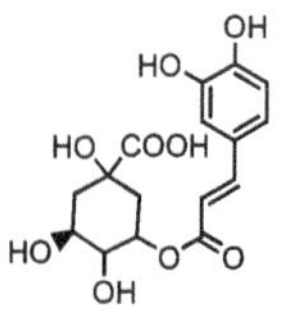

(53)

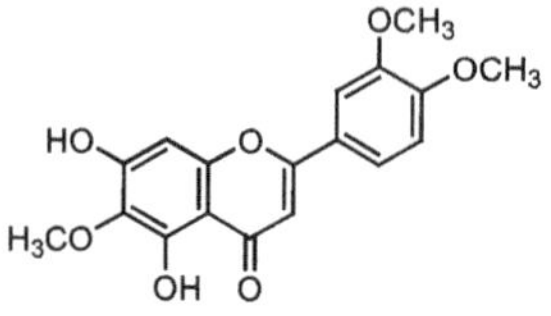

(54)

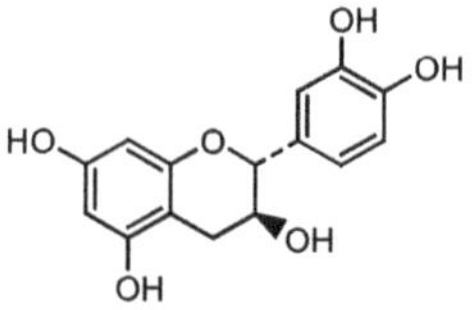

(55)

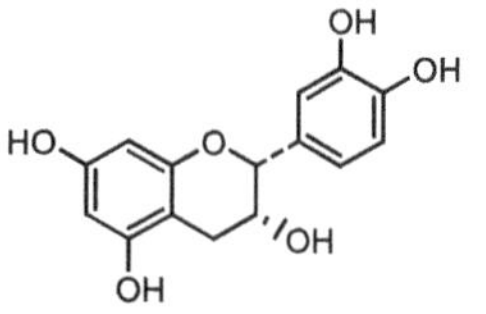

(56)

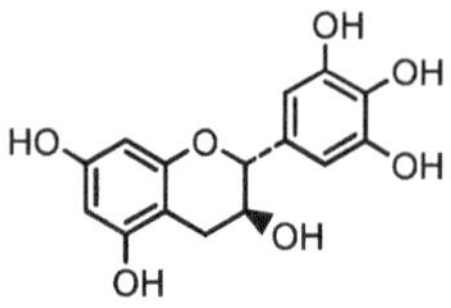

(57)

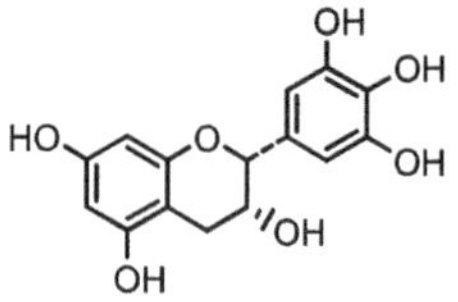

(58)

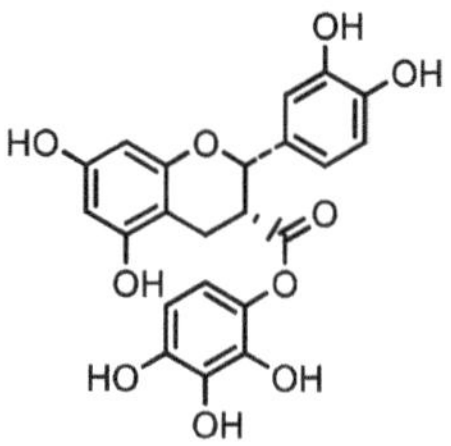

(59)

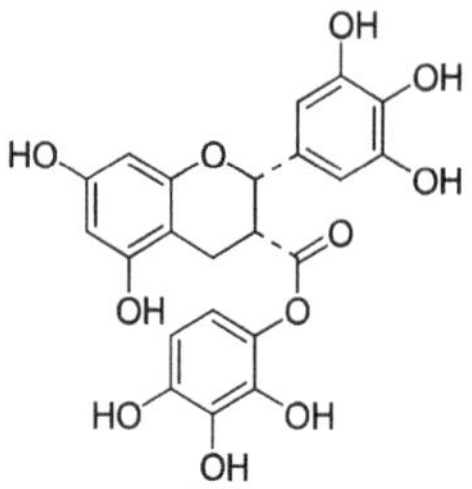

(60)

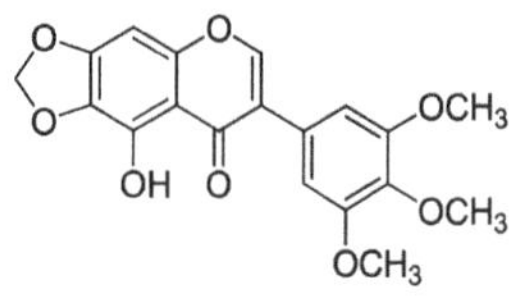

(61)

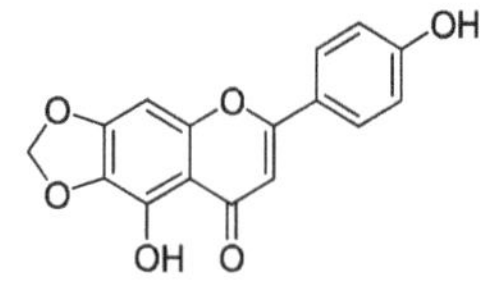

(62)

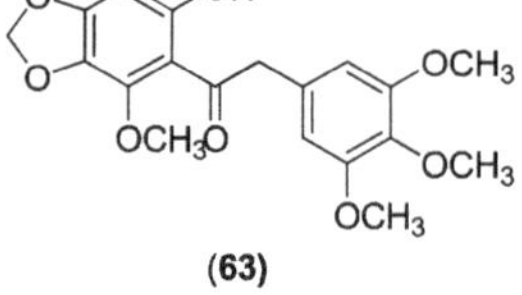

(63)

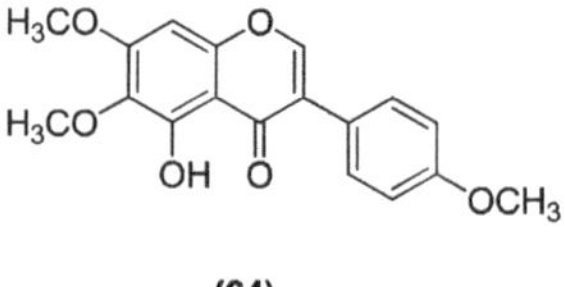

(64)

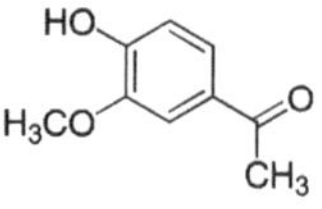

(65)

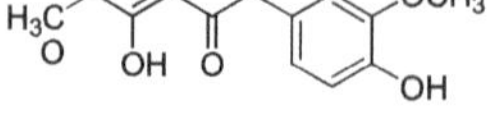

(66)

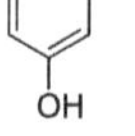

(67)

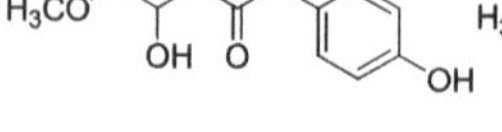

(68)

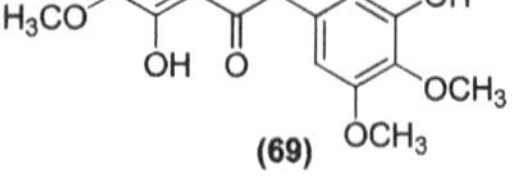

(69)

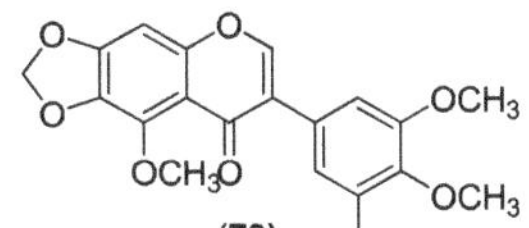

(70)

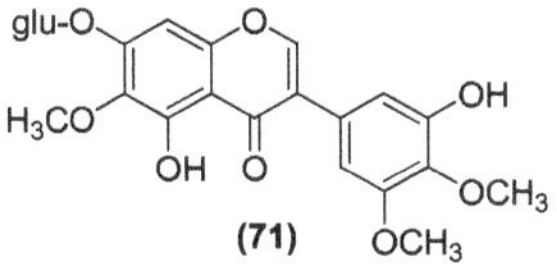

(71)

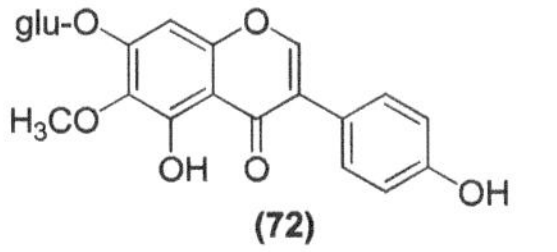

(72)

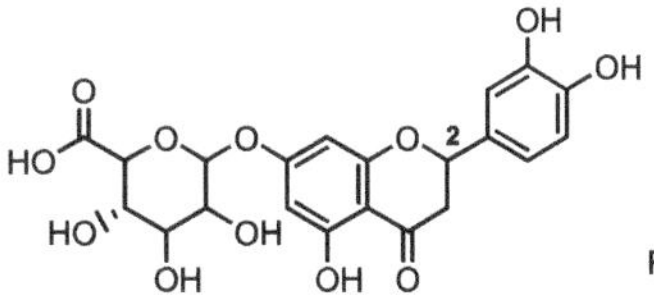

(2S)-**(73)**
(2R)-**(74)**

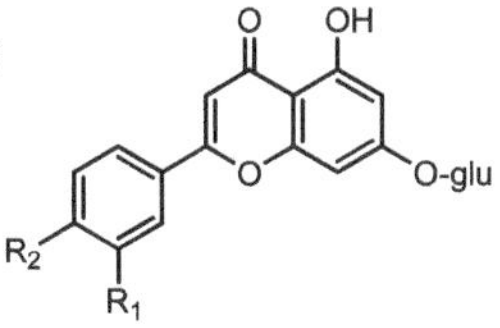

R$_1$ = H   R$_2$ = OH   **(75)**
R$_1$ = OH   R$_2$ = OCH$_3$ **(76)**

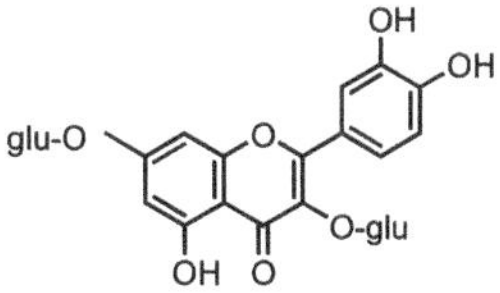

(77)

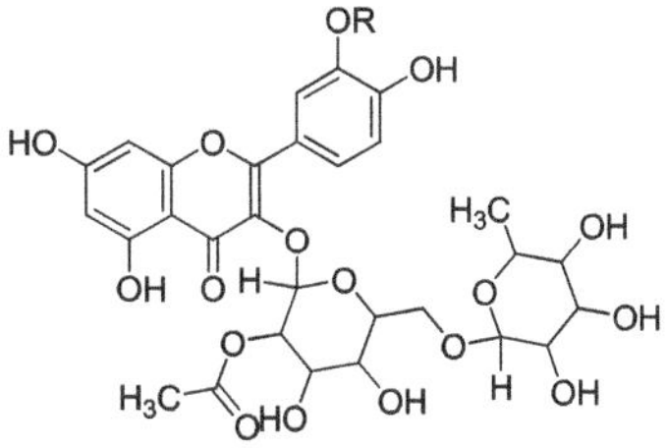

R = H   **(78)**
R = CH$_3$ **(79)**

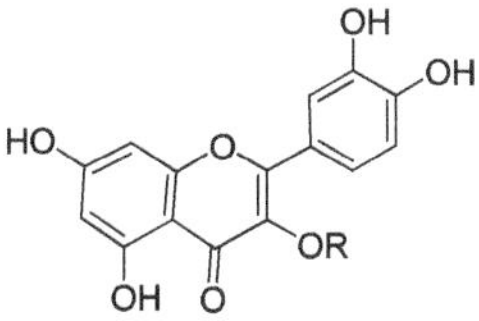

R= dirha(2→6)-gal   **(80)**
R= neohesperidoside   **(81)**

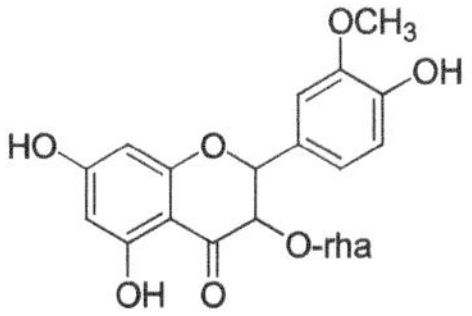

(82)

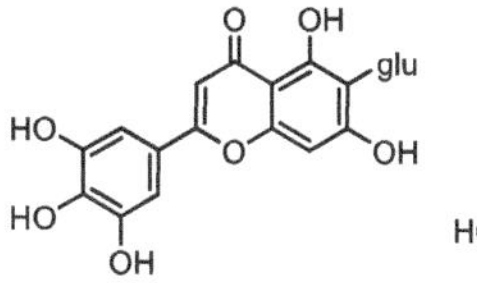

(83)

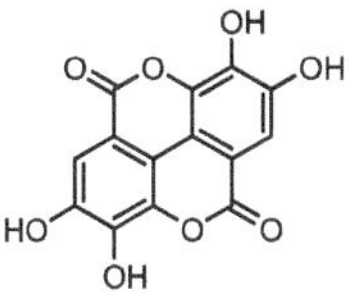

(84)

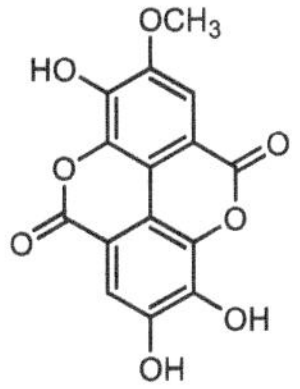

(85)

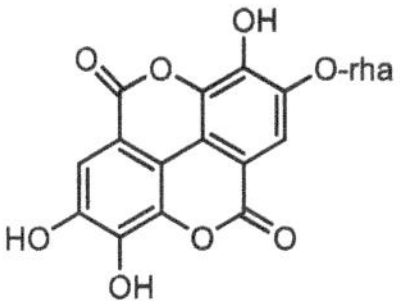

(86)

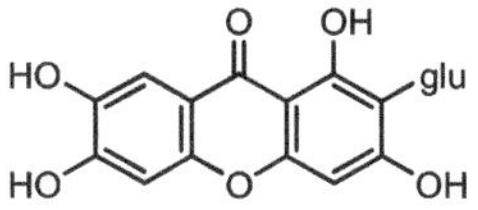

(87)

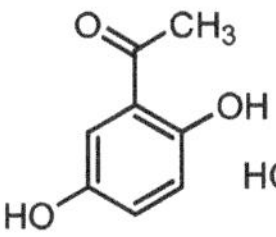

(88)

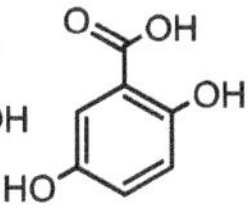

(89)

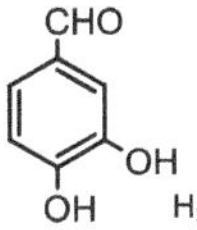

(90)

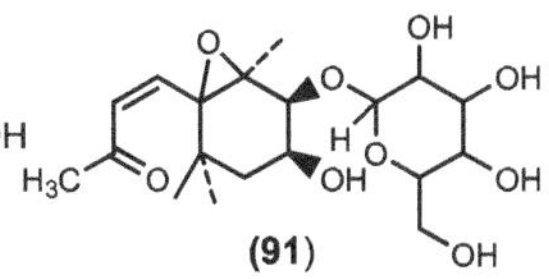

(91)

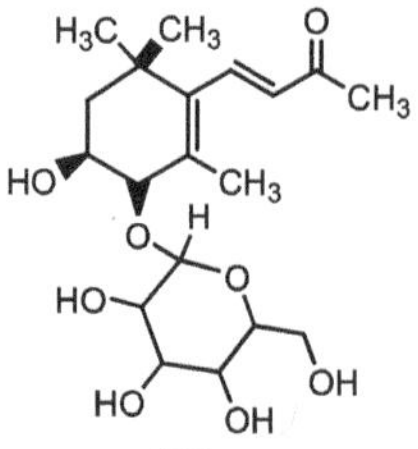

(92)

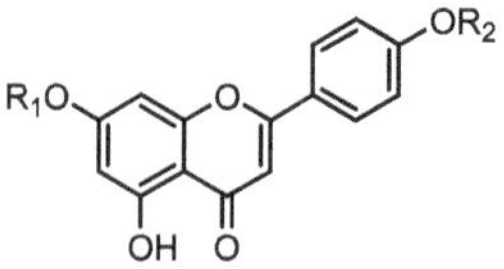

$R_1 = H$ $R_2 = H$ **(93)**
$R_1 = glu$ $R_2 = H$ **(94)**
$R_1 = H$ $R_2 = glu$ **(95)**
$R_1 = rut$ $R_2 = H$ **(96)**

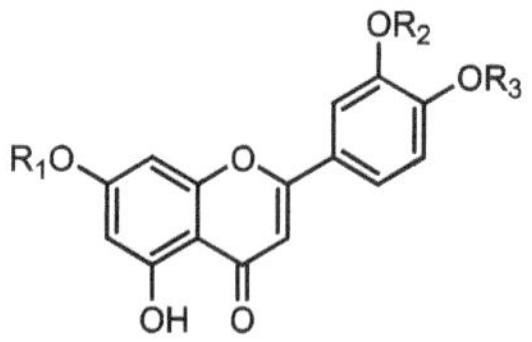

$R_1=glu$ $R_2=H$ $R_3=H$ **(97)**
$R_1=H$ $R_2=H$ $R_3=glu$ **(98)**
$R_1=rut$ $R_2=H$ $R_3=H$ **(99)**
$R_1=glu$ $R_2=CH_3$ $R_3=H$ **(100)**
$R_1=rut$ $R_2=CH_3$ $R_3=H$ **(101)**

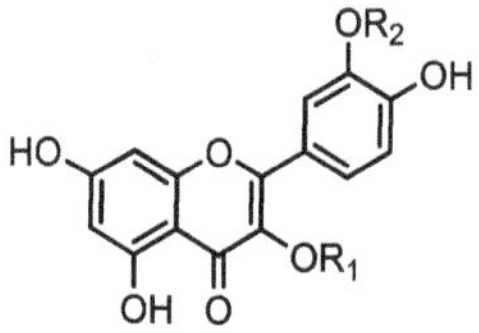

$R_1 = glu$ $R_2 = H$ **(102)**
$R_1 = rut$ $R_2 = CH_3$ **(103)**

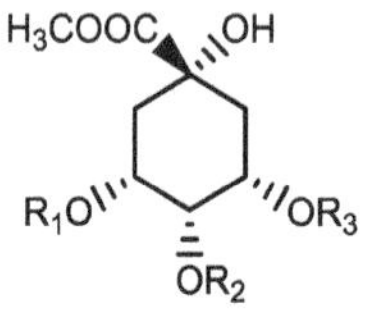

caffeoyl =

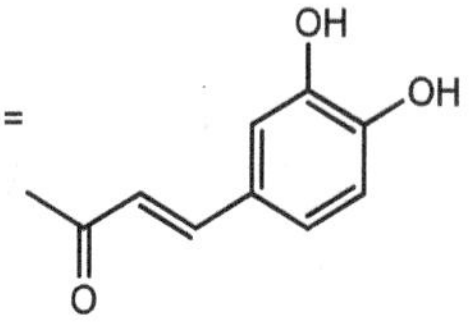

$R_1 = caffeoyl$ $R_2 = H$ $R_3 = H$ **(104)**
$R_1 = H$ $R_2 = caffeoyl$ $R_3 = H$ **(105)**
$R_1 = H$ $R_2 = H$ $R_3 = caffeoyl$ **(106)**

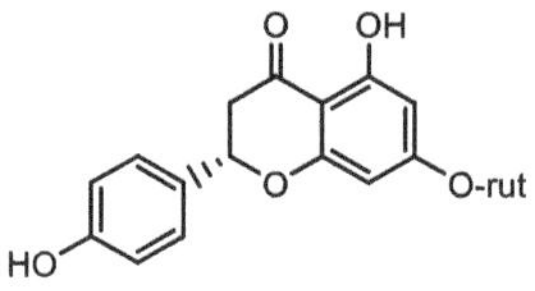

(107)

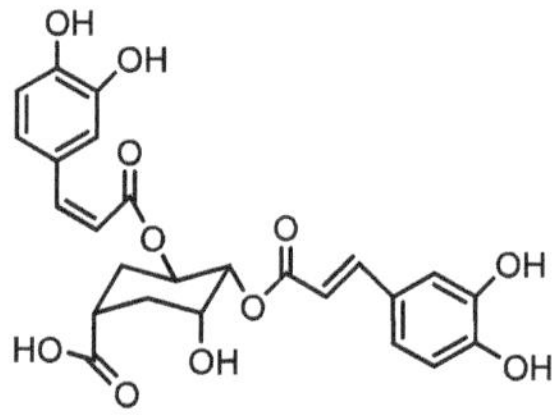

(108)

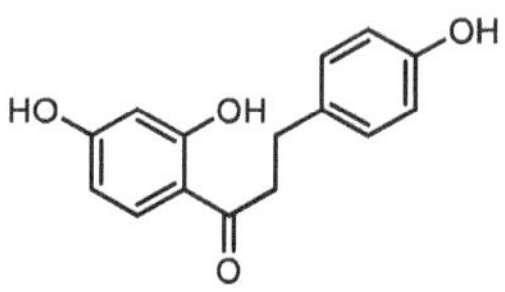

(109)

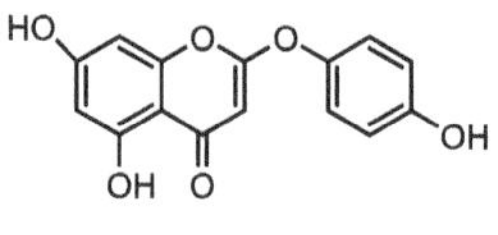

(110)

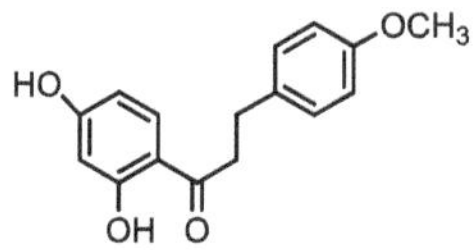

(111)

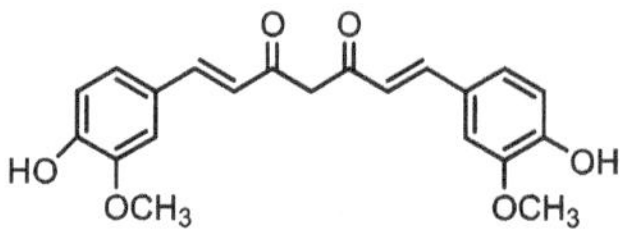

(112)

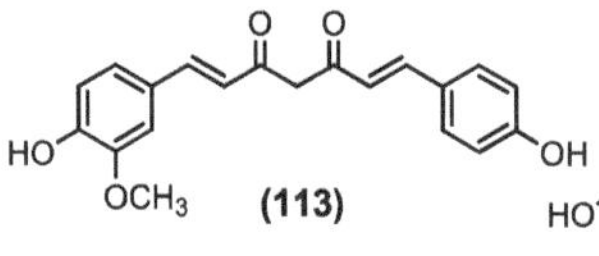

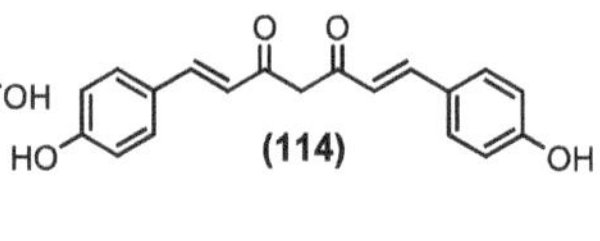

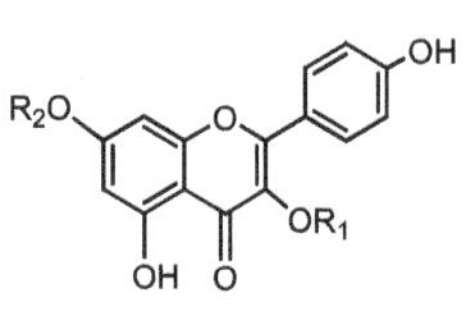

(113)

(114)

R_1	R_2	
H	H	**(115)**
gal	H	**(116)**
H	glu	**(117)**
glu	H	**(118)**
rha(1-6)glu	H	**(119)**

R_1	R_2	
rha(1-2)gln	H	**(120)**
rha(1-2)glu	H	**(121)**
glu	H	**(122)**
gln-methylester	H	**(123)**

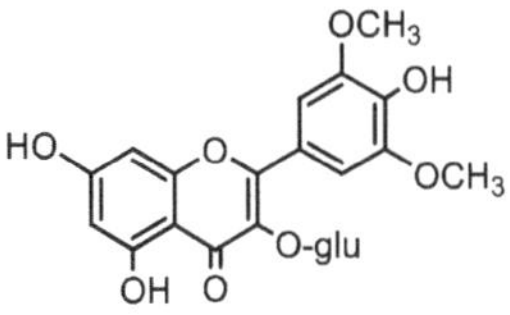

(124)

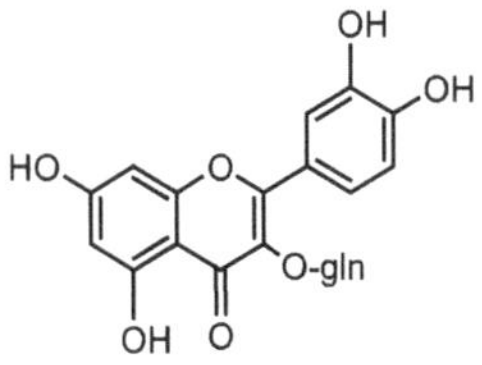

(125)

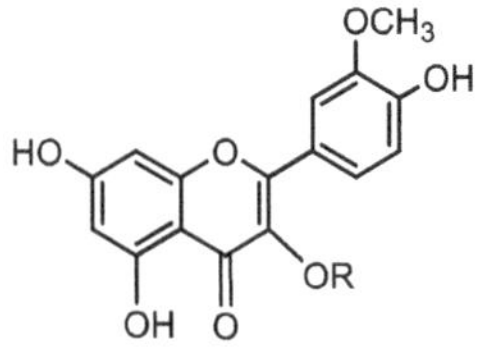

R=glu   (126)
R=rha(1-6)-glu   (127)

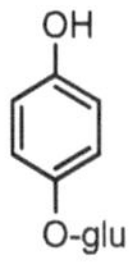

(128)

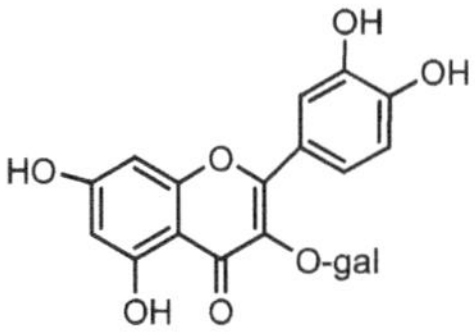

(129)

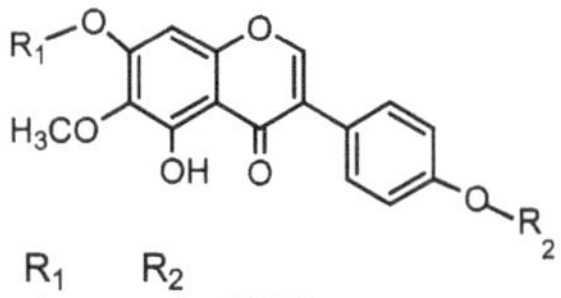

R_1	R_2	
glu	glu	(130)
H	glu	(131)

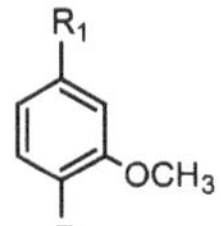

R_1	R_2	
CH_2OH	OH	(132)
$(CH_2)_2OH$	OH	(133)
CH_2COOH	OH	(134)
CH_2COOH	OCH_3	(135)
$(CH_2)_2COCH_3$	OH	(136)

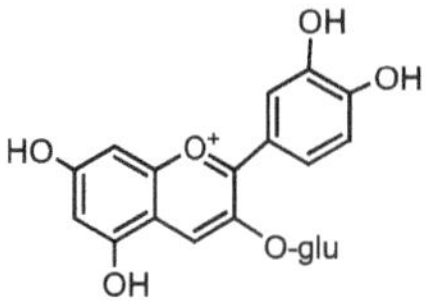

(137)

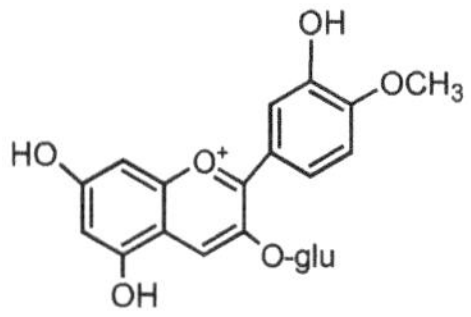

(138)

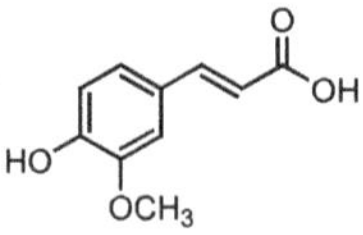

(139)

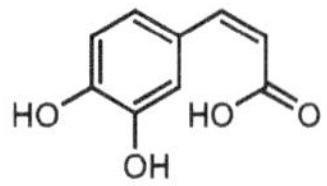

(140)

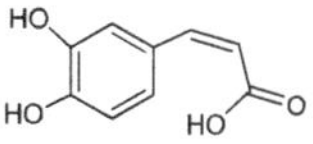

(140)

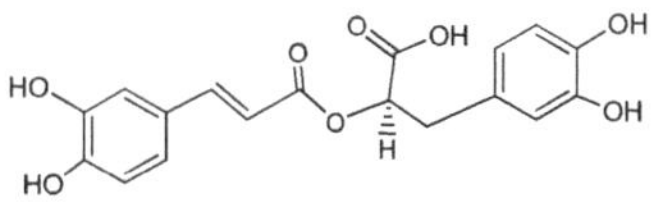

(141)

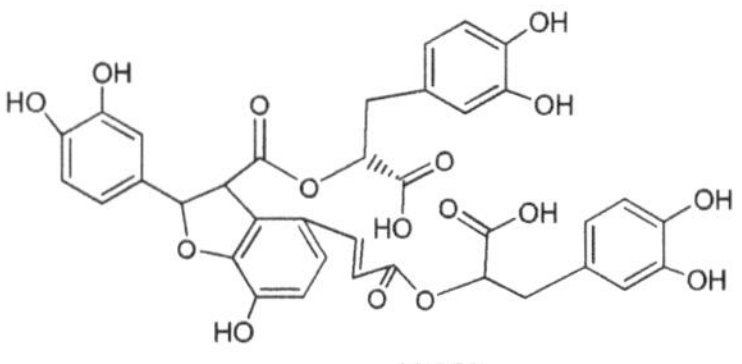

(142)

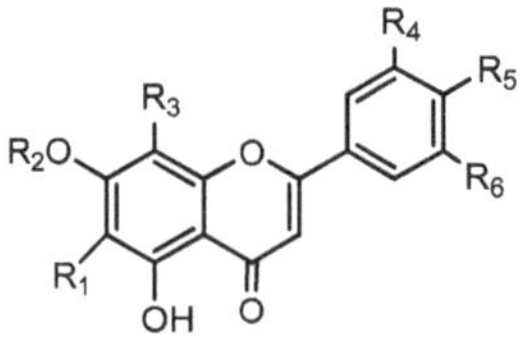

R_1	R_2	R_3	R_4	R_5	R_6	
glu	H	H	H	OH	OH	(143)
H	H	glu	H	OH	OH	(144)
H	H	glu	H	OH	H	(145)
H	glu	H	OCH_3	OCH_3	OCH_3	(147)
H	H	H	OCH_3	OH	OCH_3	(148)

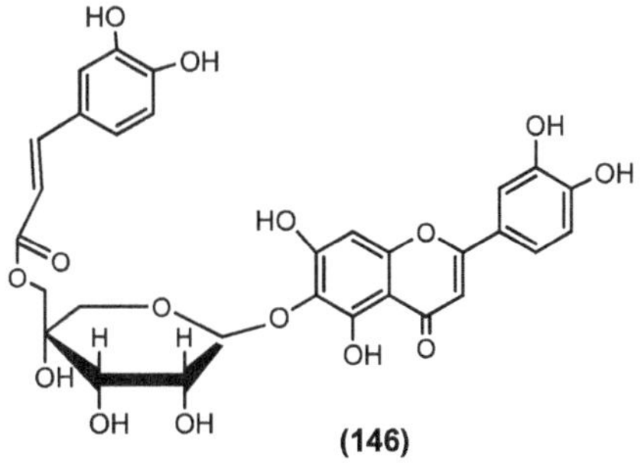

(146)

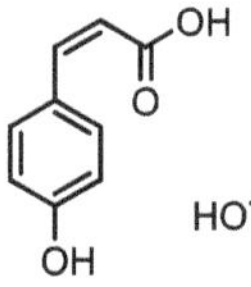

(149) 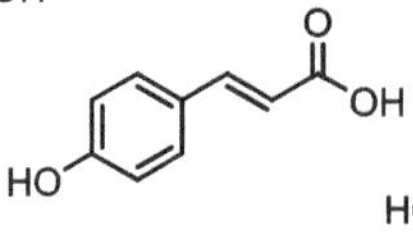   (150) 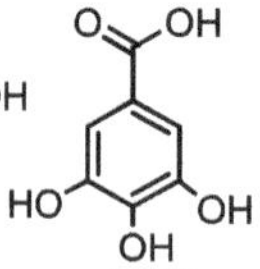   (151) 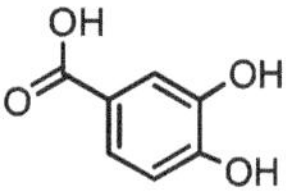   (152) 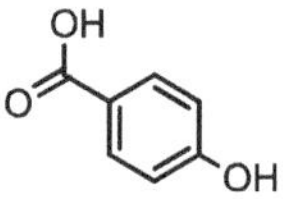   (153) 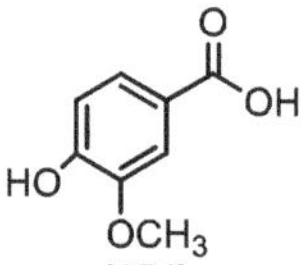   (154)

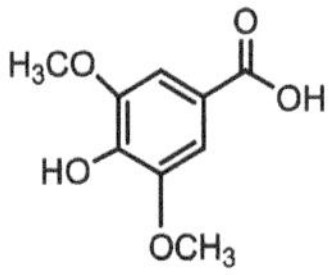

(155) 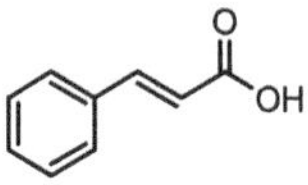   (156)

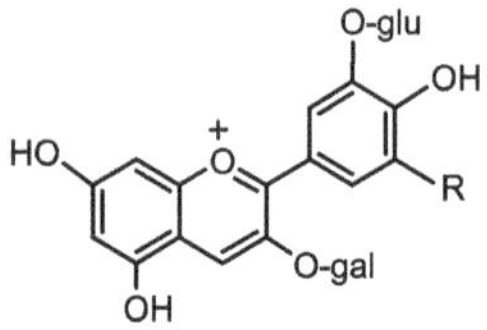

R=O-glu   (157)
R=OH   (158)

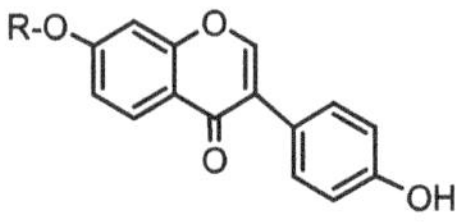

R= H   (159)
R=glu   (160)

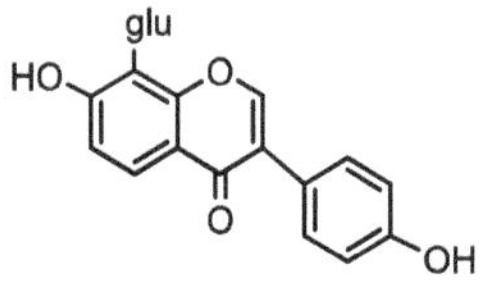

(161)

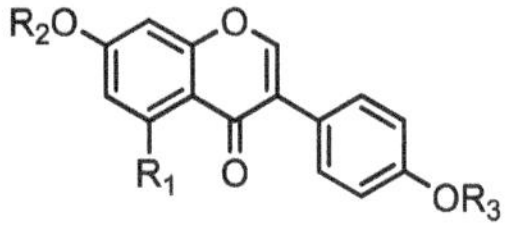

R_1=H R_2=glu R_3=CH_3 (162)
R_1=OH R_2=glu R_3=H   (163)
R_1=OH R_2=H R_3=H   (164)
R_1=H R_2=H R_3=CH_3 (165)

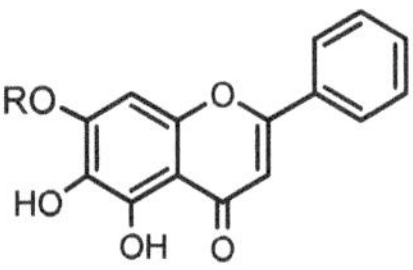

R=gln   (166)
R=H   (167)

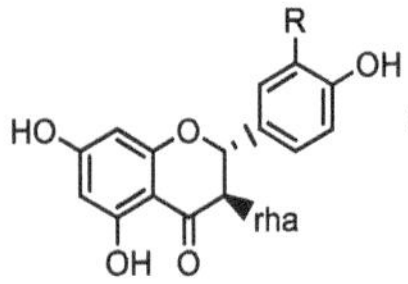

R=H   (168)
R=OH   (169)

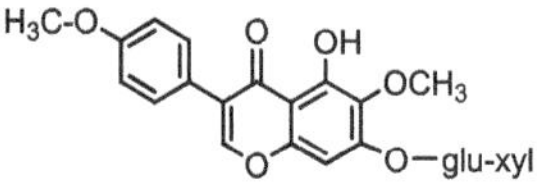

(170) 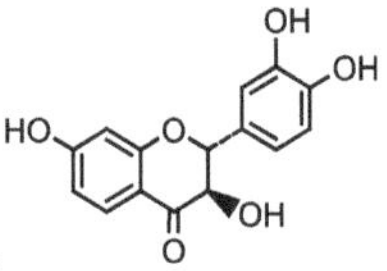   (171) 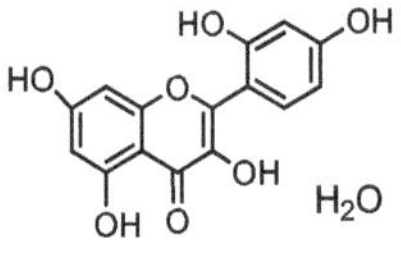   (172)

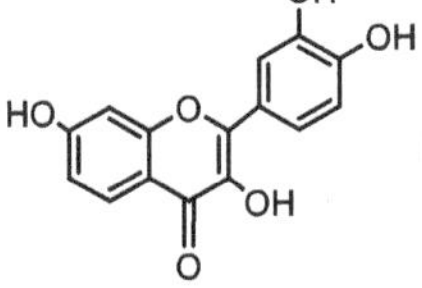

(173) 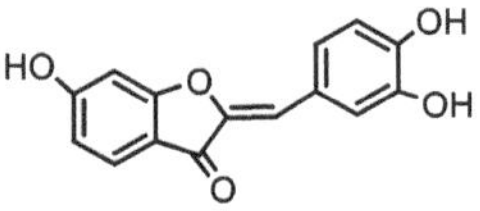   (174) 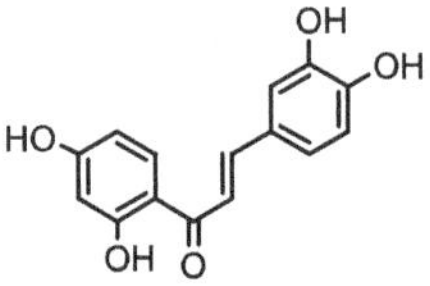   (175) 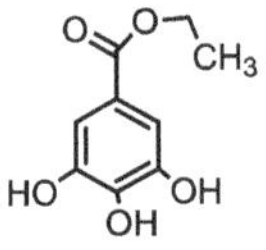   (176)

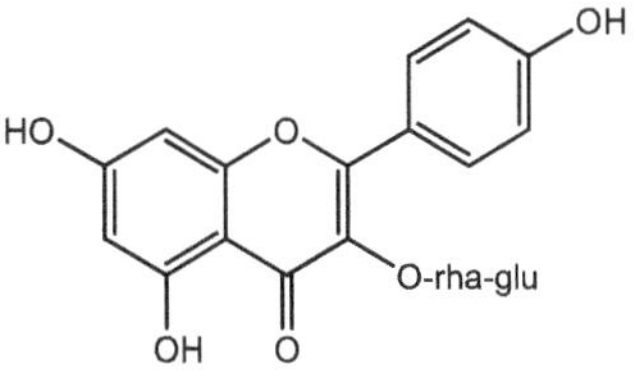

(177)

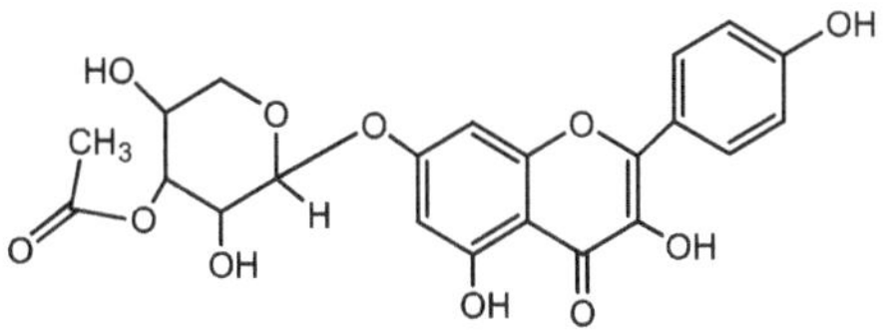

(178)

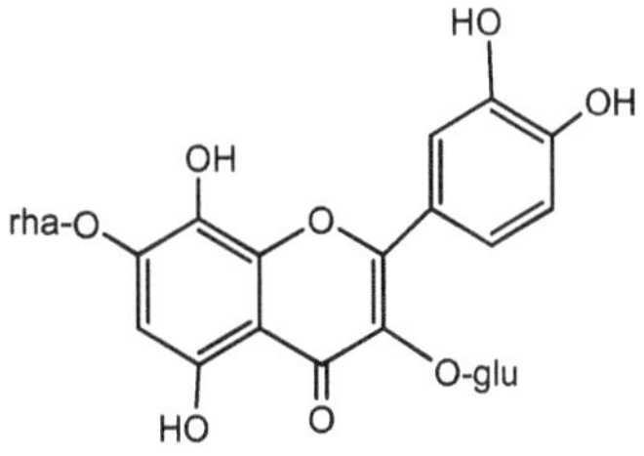

(179)

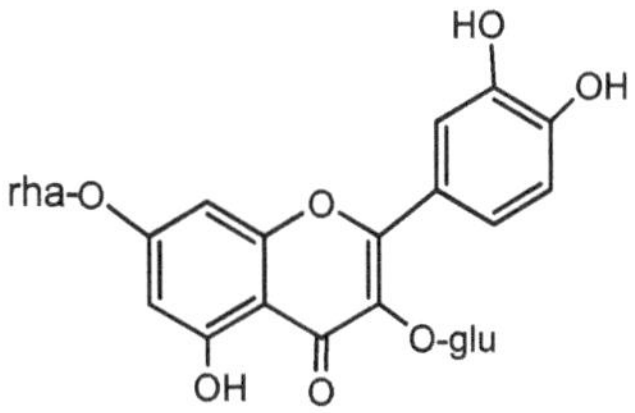

(180)

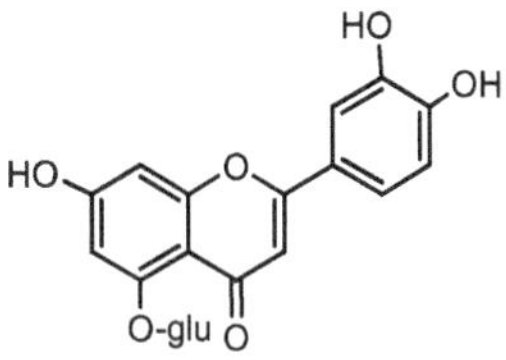

(181)

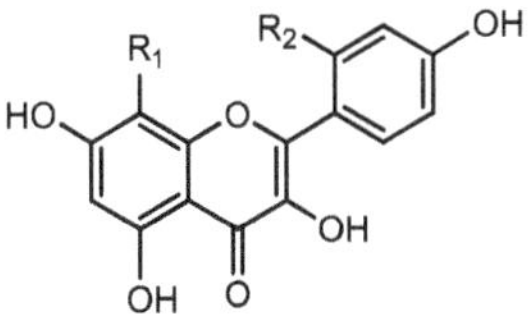

	R_1	R_2	
A	H		(182)
B	OH		(183)
B	OH		(184)

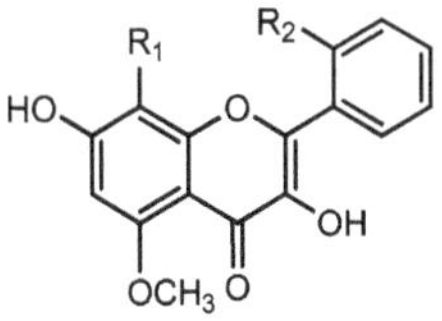

	R_1	R_2	
C	OH		(185)
B	OH		(186)
A	H		(187)

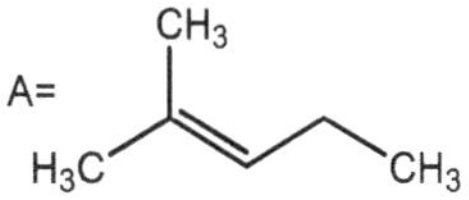

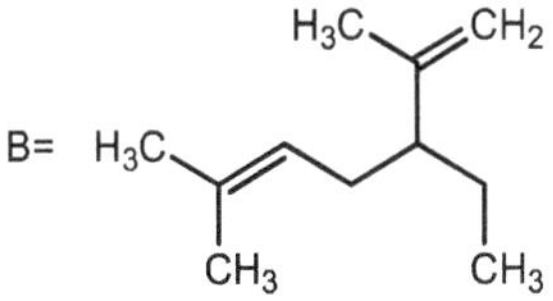

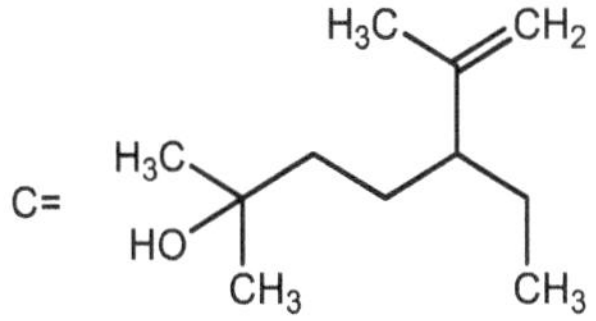

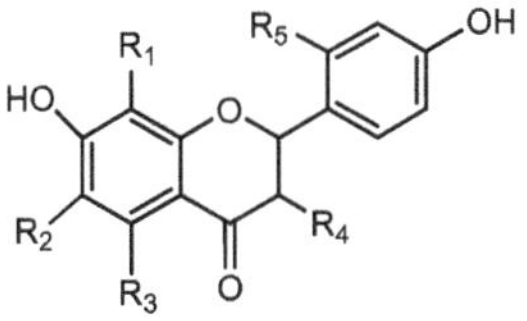

A=

B=

C=

R_1	R_2	R_3	R_4	R_5	
B	H	OH	H	OH	(188)
C	H	OCH$_3$	H	OH	(189)
B	H	OCH$_3$	H	OH	(190)
B	H	OCH$_3$	H	OCH$_3$	(191)

R_1	R_2	R_3	R_4	R_5	
A	H	OCH$_3$	OH	H	(192)
A	H	OCH$_3$	H	H	(193)
A	H	OH	H	OH	(194)
A	H	OH	H	OH	(195)

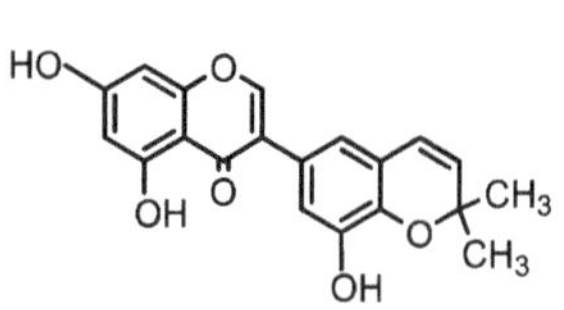

R=H   **(198)**
R=CH₃ **(199)**

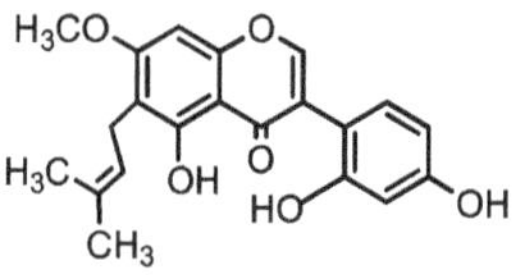

(196)

(197)

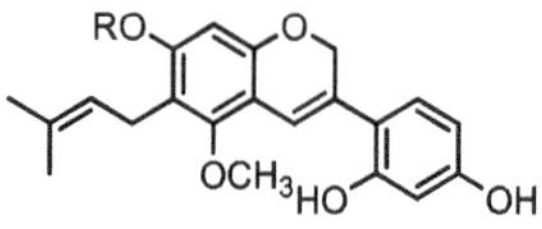

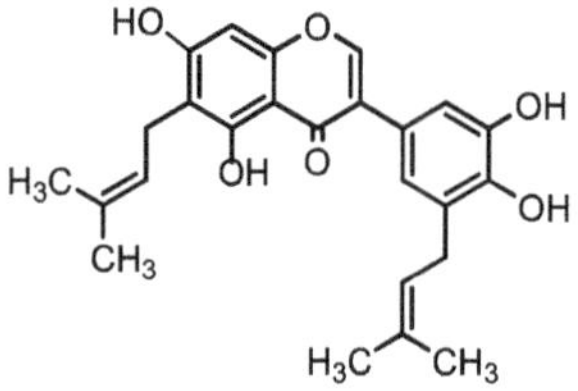

(200)

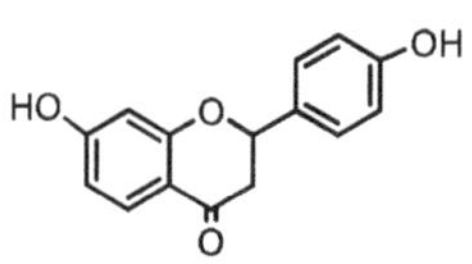

(201)

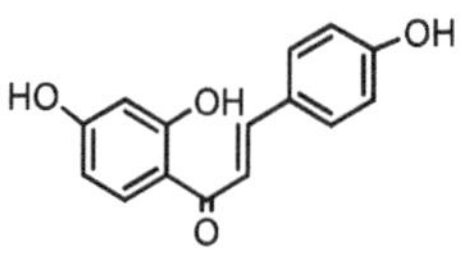

(202)

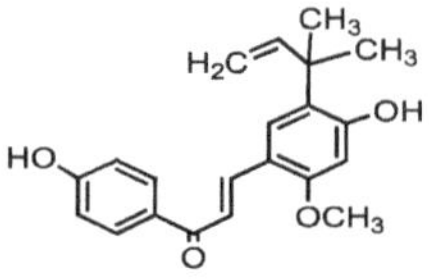

(203)

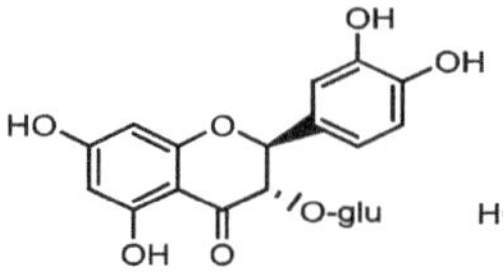

(204)

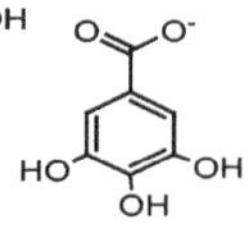

(205)

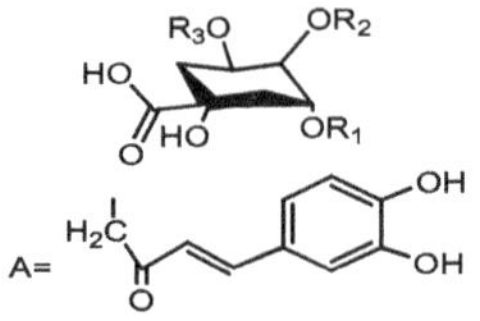

	R₁	R₂	R₃	
	A	H	A	**(206)**
	H	A	H	**(207)**
	A	H	H	**(208)**

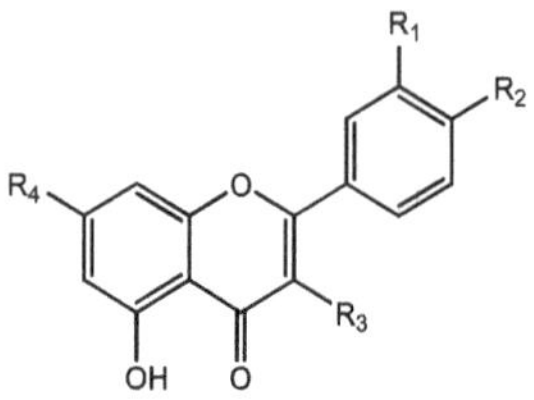

A=

R₁	R₂	R₃	R₄	
OH	OH	O-gal	OH	**(209)**
OH	OH	H	O-rut	**(210)**

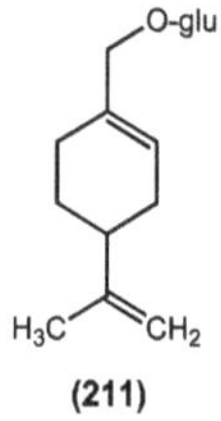

(211)

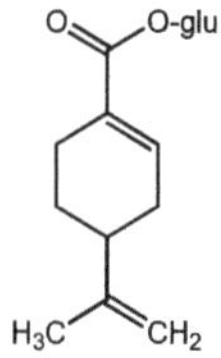

(212)

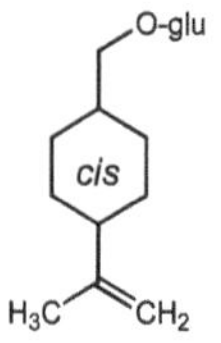

(213)

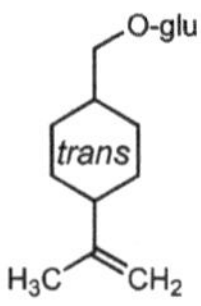

(214)

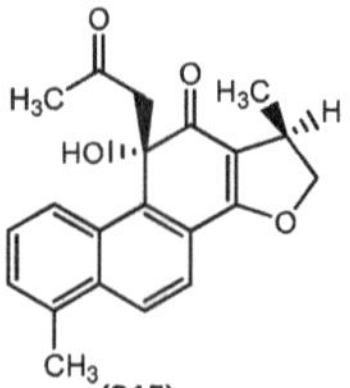

(215)

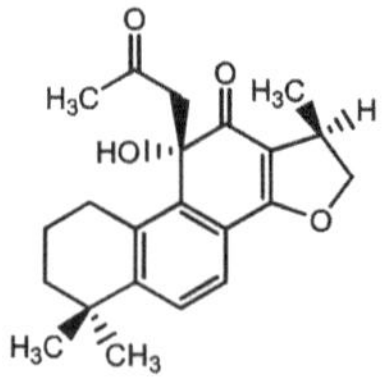

(216)

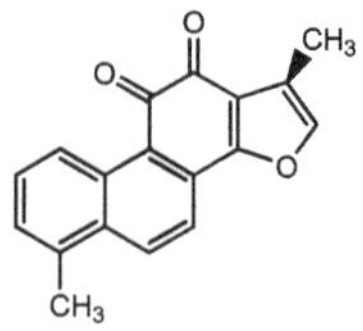

(217)

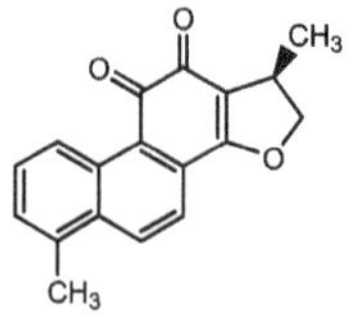

(218)

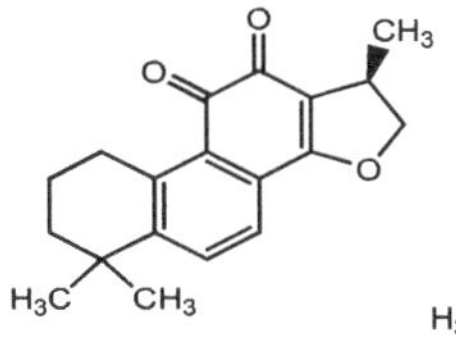

(219)

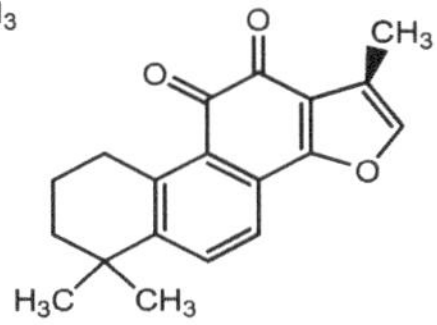

(220)

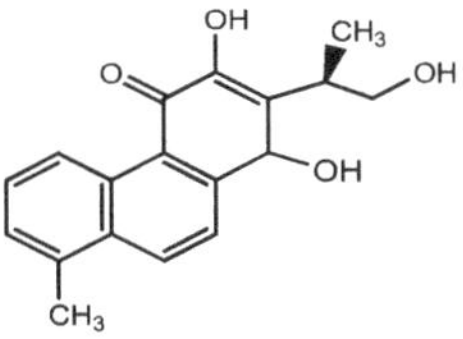

(221)

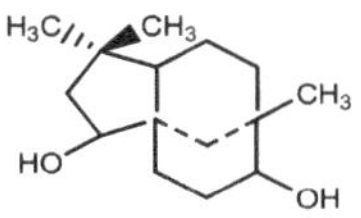

(222)

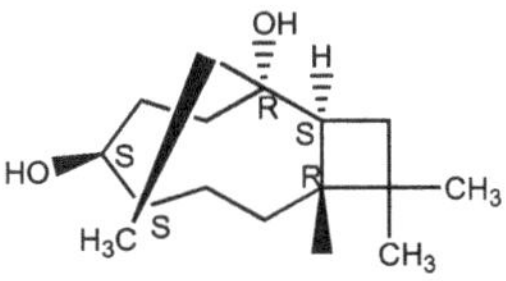

(223)

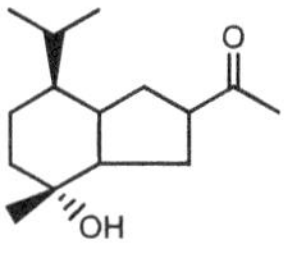

(224)

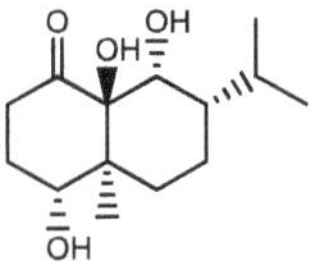

(225)

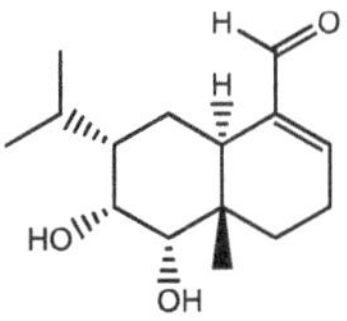

(226)

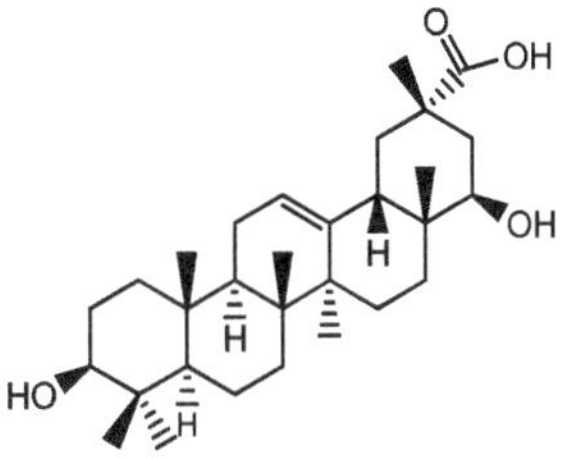

(227)

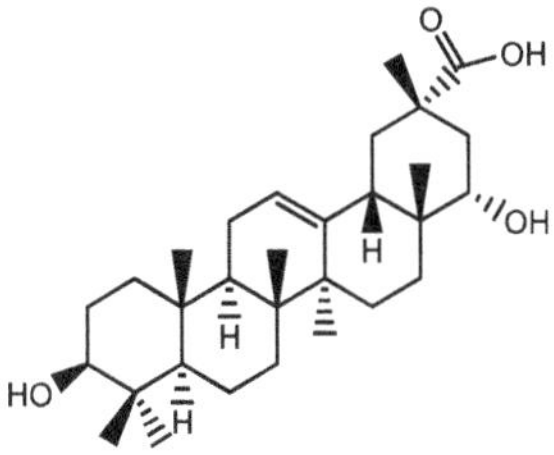

(228)

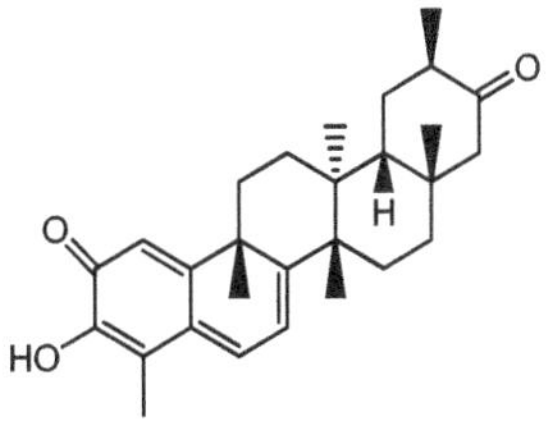

(229)

Figure 1.2 Structure of flavonoids and other phenolics with AR inhibition activity (1-208)

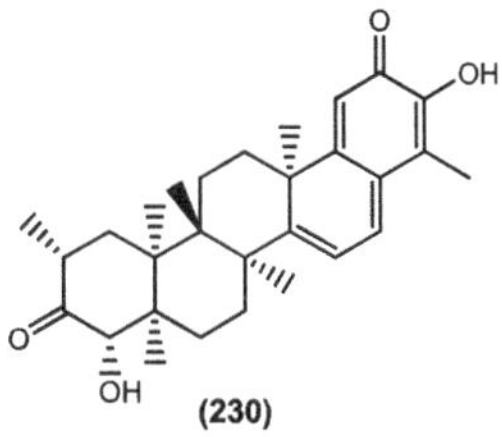

(230)

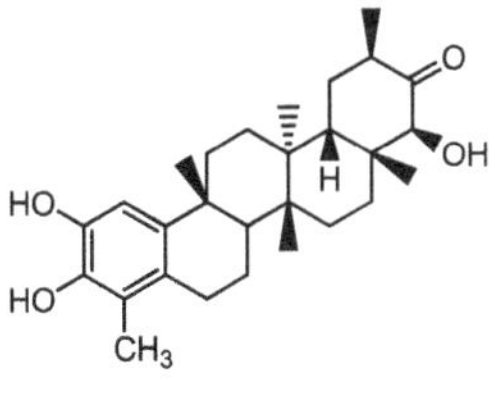

(231)

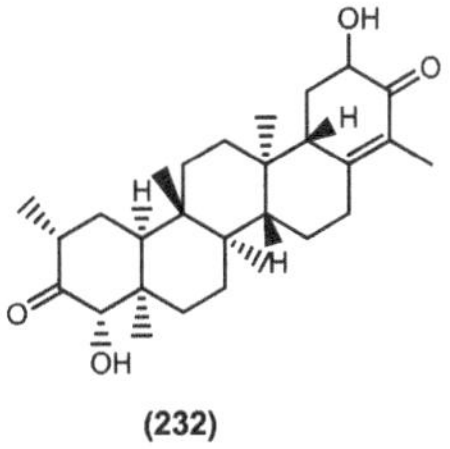

(232)

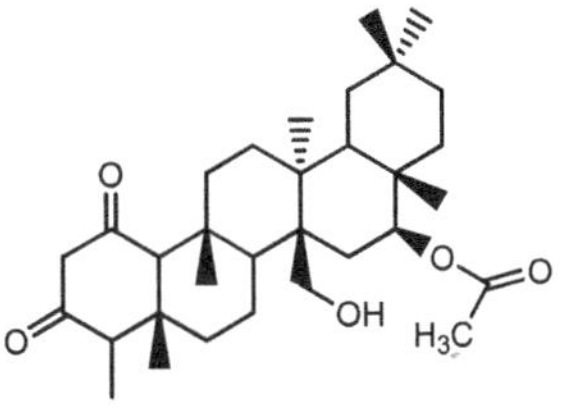

(233)

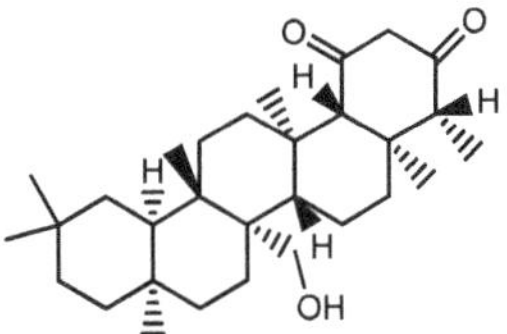

(234)

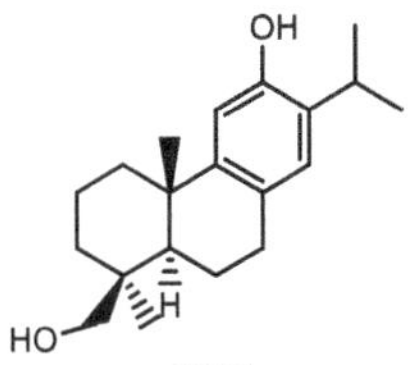

(235)

Figure 1.3 Structure of terpenoids with AR inhibition activity (209-239)

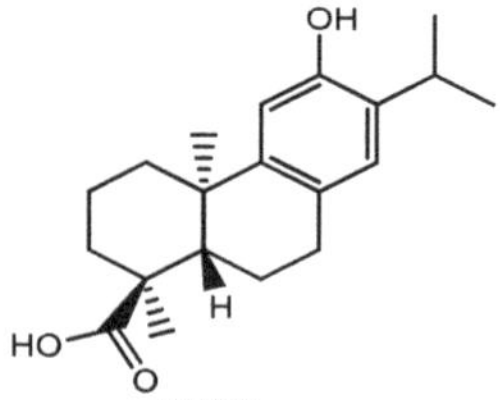

(236)

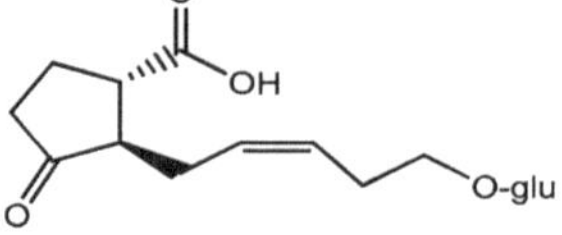

(237)

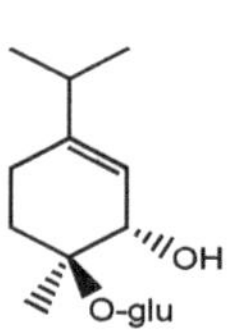

(238)

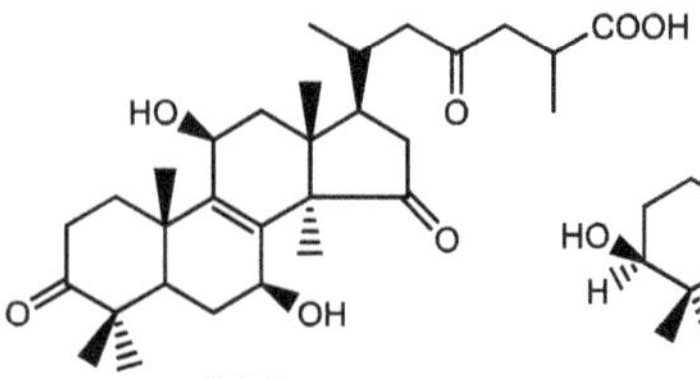

(239)

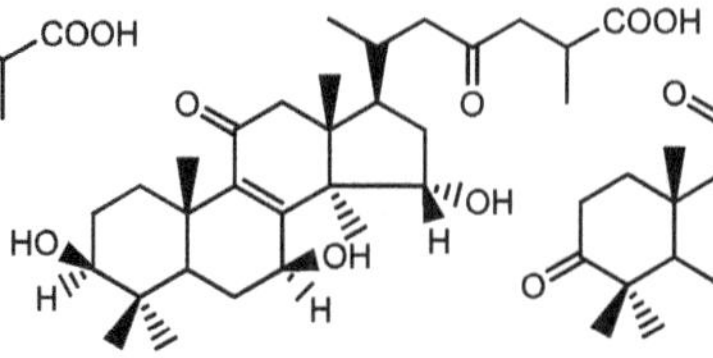

(240)

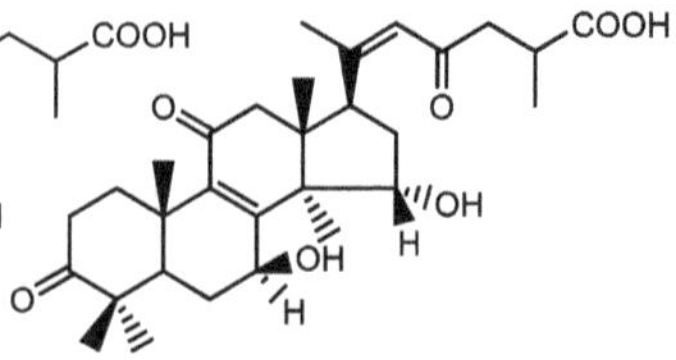

(241)

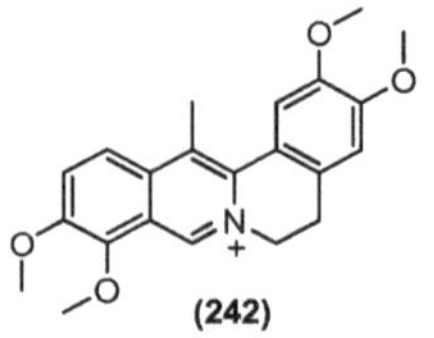

(242)

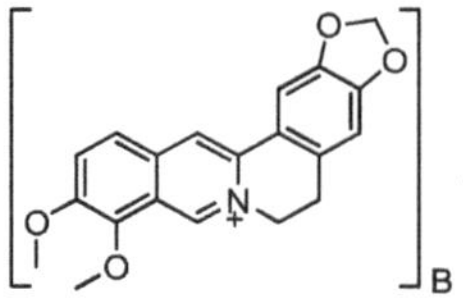

A=Cl⁻   B=1   (243)
A=SO₄⁻²   B=2   (245)
A=I⁻   B=1   (246)

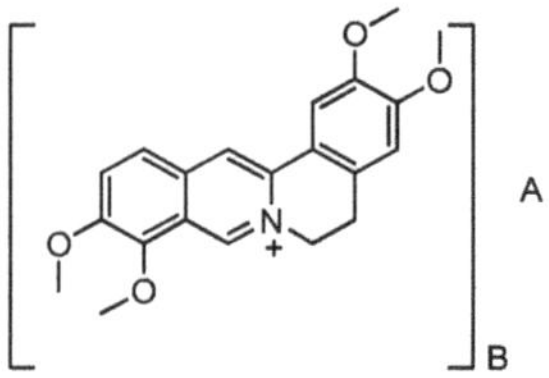

A=I⁻   B=1   (244)
A=SO₄   B=2   (247)

Figure 1.4 Structure of alkaloids with AR inhibition activity (240-246)

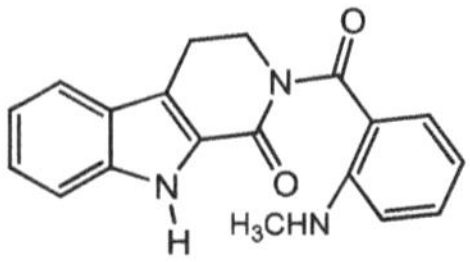

(248)

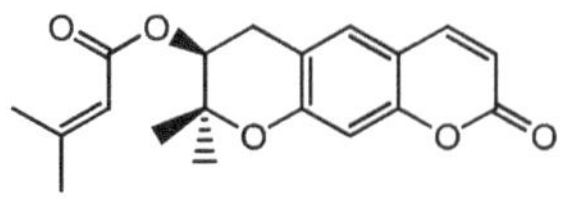

(249)

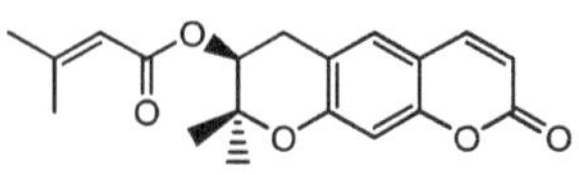

(250)

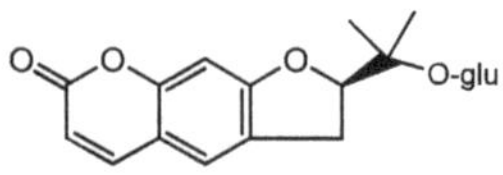

(251)

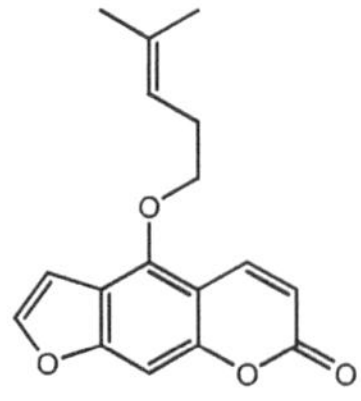

(252)

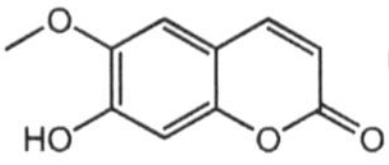

(253)

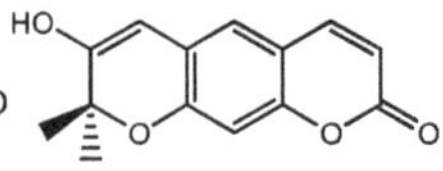

(254)

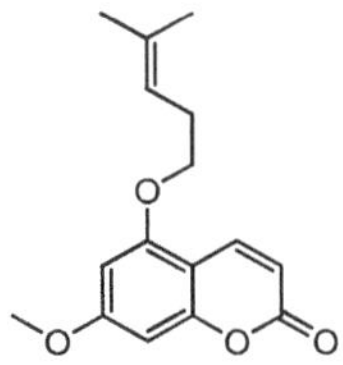

(255)

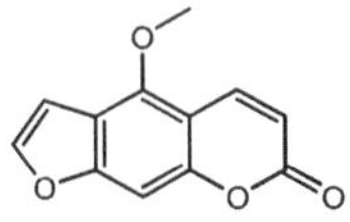

(256)

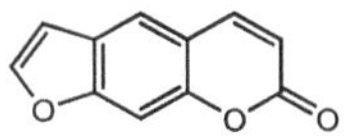

(257)

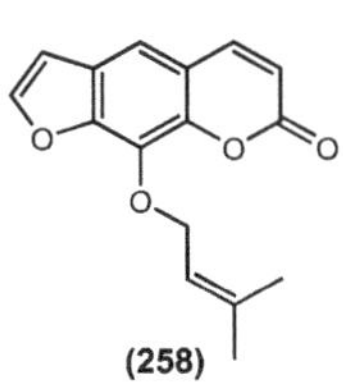

(258)

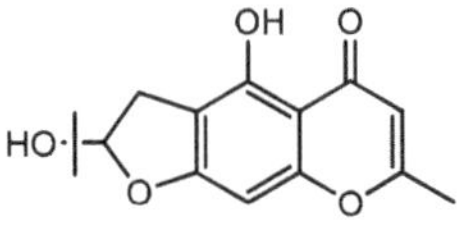

(259)

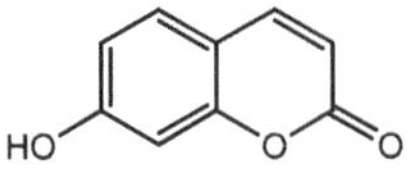

(260)

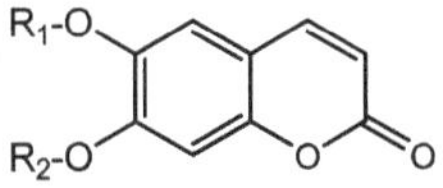

R₁   R₂
CH₃   CH₃   (261)
H   H   (262)
H   glu   (263)

Figure 1.5 Structure of coumarins with AR inhibition activity (247-262)

Figure 1.6 Structure of tannins with AR inhibition activity (263)

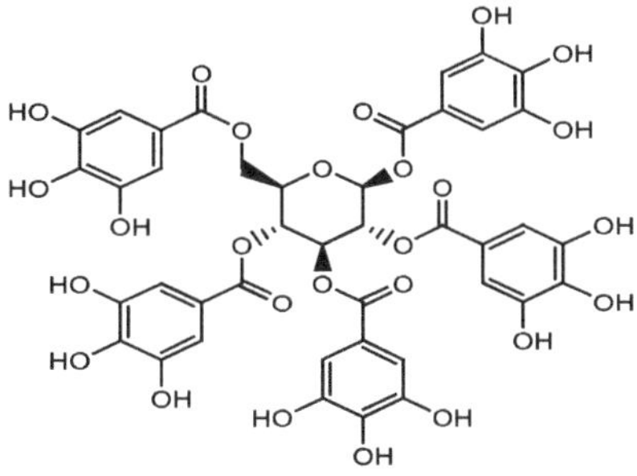

(264)

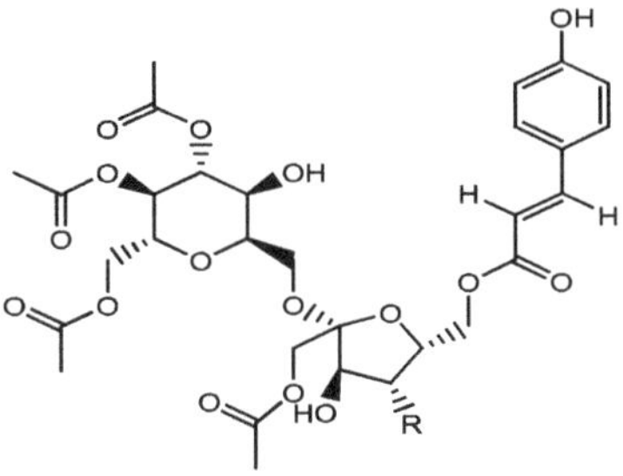

R=OCOCH₃   (265)
R=OH   (266)

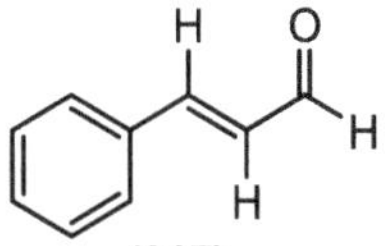

(267)

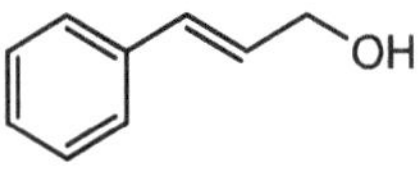

(268)

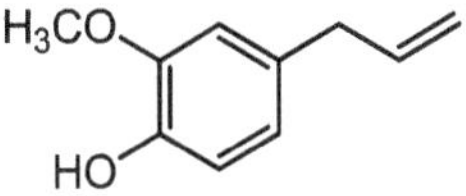

(269)

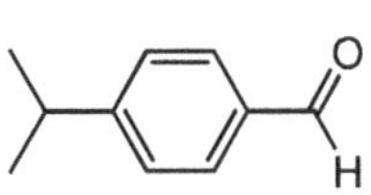

(270)

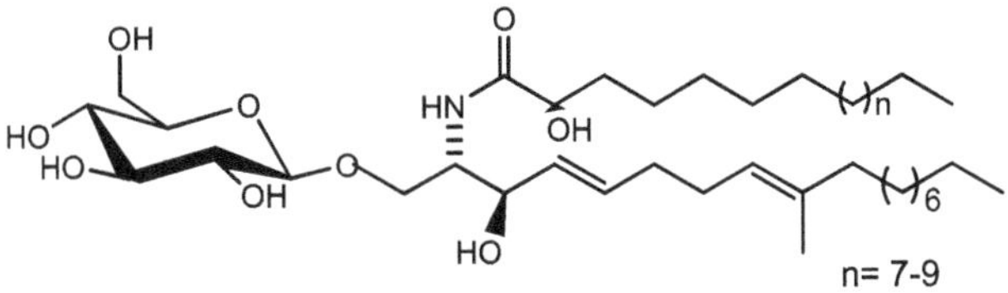

(271)

n= 7-9

Figure 1.7 Miscellaneous compounds with AR inhibition activity (264-270)

Flavonoids and other Phenolic Compounds

Flavonoids constitute one of the most characteristic classes of compounds in higher plants. They are commonly ingested from fruits and vegetables in the diet. Although flavonoids have no nutritive value, they are capable of exerting various pharmacological activities including antioxidative and AR activities. Perusal of literature reveals that a variety of flavonoids and other phenolic compounds (Figure 2) display powerful AR inhibitory activity in different *in vitro* and *in vivo* test systems.

Varma *et al.*, 1975, tested the inhibitory activities of quercetin **(1)**, rutin **(2)**, quercetrin **(3)** myrcitrin **(4)** morin **(5)**, hesperetin **(6)**, 2-carboxy-5,7-dihydroxy-4'-methoxyisoflavone **(7)** and robinin **(8)** on RLAR. The inhibioy activity of AR shown in table 1.1. It was found that quercetin **(1)**, quercitrin **(3)** and myrcitrin **(4)** are much more effective inhibitors than tetramethylene glutaric acid, previously known AR inhibitors (ARIs). They have also reported that quercetin is more potent AR inhibitor than morin, the ortho orientation of the hydroxyl group in meta and ortho of ring C rather than a meta orientation is more favorable to AR inhibitory activity. Hesperetin, in which there is the lack of double bond and the OH in ring B, and the para hydroxyl group in ring C is methylated, has much lower activity than the other aglycones. The glycoside of a flavones may be higher or lower inhibitory activity than its parent non sugar moiety, depending on the nature of the sugar moiety.

Table 1.1 Inhibition of lens AR activities by various compounds (Varma *et al.*, 1975).

Inhibitors	% inhibition at the following concentration	
	10^{-5}M	10^{-6}M
tetramethylene glutaric acid	82	35
quercetin **(1)**	83	60
rutin **(2)**	95	20
quercetrin **(3)**	95	88
myrcitrin **(4)**	100	75
morin **(5)**	75	0
hesperetin **(6)**	50	0
2-carboxy-5,7-dihydroxy-4'-methoxyisoflavone **(7)**	77	0
robinin **(8)**	56	0

Brickellia arguta belongs to family compositae and it distributed in south westeren, Mexico, and South and Central America. patuletin-3-*O*-β-D-robinoside **(9)**, patuletin-3-*O*-β-D-galactoside **(10)** and 6-methoxykaempferol-3-*O*-β-D-robinobioside **(11)**, isolated from the aqueous extract of the aerial parts of *Brickellia arguta* showed significant inhibitory activity and their potency was comparable to that of the isoquinoline derivative (alrestatin), which is regarded as one of the most promising water soluble ARIs (Rosler *et al.*, 1984). The activity of patuletin-3-*O*-β-D-robinoside **(9)** was considered to be highly significant because of its water solubility at neutral pH at pharmacologically active concentrations. The Inhibitory activity of AR shown in table 1.2.

Table 1.2 Activity of AR inhibitors (Rosler *et al.*, 1984).

Inhibitors	% inhibition at the following concentration	
	10^{-5}M	10^{-6}M
patuletin-3-*O*-β-D-robinoside **(9)**,	86	33
patuletin-3-*O*-β-D-galactoside **(10)**	84	38
6-methoxykaempferol-3-*O*-β-D-robinobioside **(11)**	63	-32
Alresatin	90	40

The AR inhibitory activity of 15 typical Lamiaceae flavonoids (Table 1.3) has been evaluated on RLAR by Tomás-Barberán *et al.* (1986). It was shown that the glycoside nepitrin **(12)**, and the aglycones sideritoflavone **(23)** and nepetin **(24)** are the active compounds with activities compare to that of quercitrin **(3)**, the positive control used in the study. Among them, there is no single compound have much potential activity than positive control. It is noteworthy that the Incorporated of a p-coumaroyl moiety in the sugar portion of monoglycosides slightly decreased their activity.

Table 1.3 Inhibitory effects of some Lamiaceae flavonoids on rat lens aldose reductase (RLAR) (Tomás-Barberán *et al.*, 1986).

Flavonoid	Common name	Source	% inhibition (10^{-5}M)
5,7,3′,4′-Tetrahydroxy-6-methoxyflavone-7-glucoside **(12)**	Nepitrin	*Rosmarinus officinalis*	72.3
5,6,7,3′,4′-Pentahydroxyflavone-7-glucoside **(13)**		*Thymus mastichina*	61.9
5,7,4′-Trihydroxy-6-methoxyflavone-7-glucoside **(14)**	Hispiduloside	*Rosmarinus officinalis*	52.0
5,7,8,3′,4′-Pentahydroxyflavone-8-glucoside **(15)**		*Sidertis mugronensis*	38.0
5,7,4′-Trihydroxy-3′-methoxyflavone-7-glucoside **(16)**		*Rosmarinus officinalis*	33.3
5,7,4′-Trihydroxy-3′-methoxyflavone-7-*p*-coumaroyl-glucoside **(17)**		*Phlomis lychnitys*	16.0

Table 1.3 *Contd...*

Flavonoid	Common name	Source	% inhibition (10^{-5}M)
3,5,7,4′-Tetrahydroxyflavone-3-*p*-coumaroyl-glucoside **(18)**	Tiliroside	*Phlomis spectabilis*	32.3
5,7,3′,4′-Tetrahydroxyflavone-7-rutinoside **(19)**		*Teucrium gnaphalodes*	61.4
5,7,3′-Trihydroxy-4′-methoxyflavone-7-rutinoside **(20)**	Diosmin	*Mentha sp.*	45.2
5,7,8,4′-Tetrahydroxy-3′-methoxyflavone-7-alosylglucoside **(21)**		*Sideritis leucantha*	24.0
5,7,3,-Trihydroxy-4′-methoxyflavone-7-neohesperidoside **(22)**	Neohesperidin	*Mentha sp.*	54.0
5,3,4′-Trihydroxy-6,7,8-trimethoxyflavone **(23)**	Sideritoflavone	*Sideritis sp.*	78.4
5,7,3′,4′-Tetrahydroxy-6-methoxyflavone**(24)**	Nepetin	*Rosmarinus officinalis*	62.0
5-Hydroxy-6,7,8, 3′,4′-pentamethoxyflavone **(25)**		*Sideritis mugronensis*	0.0
3,5,7,3′4′-Pentahydroxymethoxyflavone-3-rhamnoside **(3)**	Quercitrin	Roth	86.1

Monochasma savatieri is belonging to the family Rhinantheae, it is a perennial herb used in traditional Chinese medicine. The 70% acetone extract of the aerial parts of *M. savatierii* showed very strong inhibition of rabbit lens AR. Two phenolic glycosides: acetoside **(26)**, dehydroacetoside **(27)** along with 5 iridoid glycosides were isolated from this extract. The iridoid glycosides failed to show any activity, whilst the phenolic glycosides displayed activity (table 4) with acetoside **(26)**, exhibiting a better inhibition than the positive control, while dehydroacetoside **(27)** was not tested. The activity of acetoside **(26)** was 2.5 times more potent than baicalein, a known natural inhibitor of AR (Kodha *et al.*, 1989).

Table 1.4 Activity of AR inhibitors (Kodha *et al.*, 1989).

Compounds	IC_{50} (M)
acetoside **(26),**	3.90×10^{-7}
dehydroacetoside **(27)**	Not tested
Demethylmussaenoside	6.14×10^{-5}
7-*O*-acetyl-8-epi-loganic acid	5.60×10^{-5}
Catalpol	-------
Bartisioside	--------
Aucubin	--------
Baicalein	9.80×10^{-7}

Traditionally in Japan, some kampo medicines have been prescribed for the alleviation of subjective symptoms of diabetic neuropathy. Which contain Glycyrrhizae radix (GR *Glycyrrhizae uralensis* Fischer)) and Paeoniae radix (PR *Paeonia lactiflora* Pallas)) have long been used for the treatment of diabetic neuropathy. Kaoru *et al.,* 1989, isolates the nine compounds from the boiled water extract of GR and PR. Among the seven of GU compounds, GU-2 (isoliquiritin) was the most potent inhibitor of rat lens aldose reductase (RLAR) by inhibiting 86% at the concentration of 1.0 µg/mL (Table 1.5). The IC_{55} of GU-2 was 7.2×10^{-7}M. Compounds PR-1 and PR-2 of PR inhibited RLAR by 77.6% and 61.0%, respectively, at the concentrations of 1 µg/mL. The IC_{50} of PR-1 on RLAR was determined to be 6.3×10^{-7} M.

Table 1.5 RLAR Inhibitiory ativity of kampo medicines, (Kaoru et al., 1989).

Compounds	%inhibition (µg/mL)	
	1.0	0.1
Liquiritin	23.5	0
Isoliquiritin	75.4	34.6
liquiritigenin	62.7	12.0
licuraside	74.3	22.1
Naringenin-4-*0*-β-D-glucoside	19.3	0.5
1,2,3,6-tetra-*O*-galloyl-3-β-D-glucose	77.6	3.0
1,2,3,4, 6-penta-*O*-galloyl-3-β-D-glucose	61.0	2.9

3,3',4-Tri-O-methylellagic acid 4'-sulfate potassium salt was isolated from a Mexican herb "Sinfito" (*Potentilla candicans*) as a potent AR inhibitory active constituent. 3,3',4-Tri-O-methylellagic acid 4'-sulfate potassium salt was more potent (IC50 = $8.0 \times 10(-8)$ M) than ellagic acid, which is one of the natural inhibitors of AR.

Anacardium occidentale belongs to the family Anarcardiaceae, Toyomizu et al., 1993 isolated the sixteen compounds from the methanolic extracts of *Anacardium occidentale* and evalavuvated the BLAR activity. Among the tested against BLAR, 6-Pentadecatrienlysalicylic acid is the strongest inhibitor followed by 5-pentadecadienyl, and 5-pentadecatrielnylresorcinol (Table 1.6).

Table 1.6 AR Inhibitiory ativity of compounds isolated from the nuts of *Anacardium occidentale* at a concentration of 100 Mm, (Toyomizu et al., 1993).

Compounds	IC_{50}(M)
1,6-pentadecylsalicylic acid	100.4
6-[8(Z)-pentadeccnyl] salicylic acid;	40.4
6-18(Z), 11 (Z)-pentadecadienyl] salicylic acid;	49.3

Table 1.6 *Contd...*

Compounds	$IC_{50}(M)$
6-[8(Z),11 (Z), 14-pentadecatrienyll] salicylic acid;	20.4
3-pentadecylphenol; 6, 3-[8(Z)-pentadecenyll phenol;	>328.4
3-[8(Z)-pentadecenyl] phenol	>330.6
3-[8(Z),11 (Z)-pentadecadienyl] phenol;	332.8
3-18(Z), 11(Z), 14-pentadecatrienyll phenol;	180.9
2-methyl-5-pentadecyl resorcinol;	NT
2-methyl-5[8(Z)-pentadecenyl] resorcinol;	300.7
2-methyl-5[8(Z), 11 (Z)-pentadecadienyll resorcinol;	118.0
2-methyl-5[8(Z), ll (Z). 14-pentadecatrienyll resorcinol;	115.7
5-pentadecyl resorcinol;	312.0
5-[8(Z)-pentadecenyl]-resorcinol;	28.3
5-[8(Z), 1l(Z)-pentadecadienyll resorcinol;	28.4
5-[8(Z),11*(Z)*,14-pentadecatrienyl] resorcinol.	57.2

rhamnocitrin, Capillarisin **(28)** and cirsimaritin **(29)** isolated from the ethyl acetate extract of *Artemisa capillaris* exhibited a potent inhibitory effect on bovine lens AR (BLAR). Capillarisin **(28)** was found to be much more potent than the others with activity exceeding those of the positive control quercetin and quercitrin Shown in Table 1.7 (Okada *et al.*, 1995).

Table 1.7 Inhibitory effect of the test compound on BLAR (Okada *et al.*, 1995).

Compounds	Conc(μg/ml)	%inhibition	IC_{50} (M)
rhamnocitrin	10	21	-----
Capillarisin (28)	1	89	0.22
cirsimaritin (29)	10	91	1.6
quercetin	10	88	0.84
Quercitrin	3	81	0.5

Haraguchi *et al.* (1996) isolated nine flavonoids namely, quercetin **(1)**, 3-sulfate quercetin **(30)**, isorhamnetin **(31)**, percicarin **(32)**, isorhamnetin-3,7-disulfate **(33)**, rhamnazin **(34)**, rhamnazin-3-sulfate **(35)**, isoquercitrin **(36)**, and tamarixetin-3-glucoside 7-sulfate **(37)** from the leaves of *Polygonum hydropiper*. All of them showed varying degrees of inhibitory effect on PL (porcine lens) AR (Table 1.8). But, isorhamnetin-3,7-disulfate **(33)** was the most potent with an IC_{50} value of 1.8 μM. Kinetic analysis proved that isorhamnetin-3, 7-disulfate **(33)** exhibited noncompetitive inhibition against both *dl*-glyceraldehyde and NADPH. In this study, also explain about the importance of sulfonation and methylated derivate of flavonoids, if removal of one or both sulfate moiety from isorhamnetin-3, 7-disulfate **(33)** abolish the AR inhibitory activity. Similarly, methyalation of quercetin **(1)**, 3-sulfate quercetin **(30)**, isorhamnetin (31) at C-3' caused a decrease in the inhibitory activity. And other hand, sulfonation at

7th position and methylation at 3' to isoquercitrin (**36**), to form tamarixetin-3-glucoside 7-sulfate (**37**) with greater PL inhibitory activity.

Table 1.8 Effect of flavonoids isolated from the leaves of *Polygonum hydropiper* PLAR Haraguchi *et al.* (1996). (Inhibitory activity as expressed as the mean of 50% inhibitory concentration of triplicate determination).

Compounds	IC_{50}
quercetin (1)	50.1
3-sulfate quercetin (30)	50.9
isorhamnetin (31)	>95.0
percicarin (32)	69.0
isorhamnetin-3,7-disulfate (33)	1.8
rhamnazin (34)	>91.0
rhamnazin-3-sulfate (35)	30.1
isoquercitrin (36)	16.0
tamarixetin-3-glucoside 7-sulfate (37)	5.0

Engelhardtia chrysolepis is belongs to family juglandaceae, is a subtropical tree grown in Guangdong, Guangxi, and China. Dried leaves of this plant are used as a sweet tea to prevent obesity and are used in folk medicine as an antifebrite and anodyne. The dihydroflavonol, taxifolin (**38**) and its rhammnoside, astilbin (**39**) isolated from the leaves of the *E. chrysolepis* have been reported to inhibit both HRAR and RLAR. In this study It was observed that the aglycone possesses less activity than the glycoside on RLAR assay, whilst the activity of the aglycone was better than its rhamnoside on HRAR (Table 1.9) (Haraguchi *et al.*, 1997).

Table 1.9 Inhibitory effect of taxifolin and astilbin on both HRAR and RLAR (Haraguchi *et al.*, 1997).

Compounds	Conc(μg/mL)	RLAR %inhibition	HRAR %inhibition
astilbin (39)	10	63	30
	6.1	50	15
taxifolin (38)	10	55	60
	6.1	18	35

In Brazil, the leaves of *Myrcia multiflora* (LAM.) DC. Which is belonging to the family Myrtaceae, which is widely distributed in Brazil and Paraguay. Leaves of *M. multiflora* are used for the treatment of diabetes. Phytochemical analysis of the ethyl acetate-soluble portion of the methanolic leaf extracts of the plant by Yoshikawa *et al.* (1998) resulted in the isolation of secondary metabolites including the flavanone glucosides myrciaacitrin 1 (**40**) and myrciaacitrin 2 (**41**); the flavonol glucosides myricitrin (**42**), mearnsitrin (**43**), quercitrin (**3**) desmanthin-1 (**44**) and guaijaverin **(45)**; and the acetophenone glucosides myrciaphenone A **(46)** and myrciaphenone B **(47).** All the principal constituents including myrciacetin **(48),** the aglycone of the major constituent myrciaacitrin 1 **(40)** showed potent inhibitory activity on RLAR enzyme. But, desmanthin-1 **(44)** (IC_{50} = 8.2 X 10^{-8} M) was the most potent of all with activity equivalent to that of the commercial synthetic AR inhibitor, epalrestat (Table 1.10).

Table 1.10 Inhibitory activity on RLAR enzyme. (Yoshikawa *et al.*, 1998)

Compounds	$IC_{50}(M)$
myrciaacitrin 1 (40)	3.2×10^{-6}
myrciaacitrin 2 (41)	1.5×10^{-5}
myricitrin (42)	3.8×10^{-5}
mearnsitrin (43)	1.4×10^{-6}
quercitrin (3)	1.5×10^{-7}
desmanthin-1 (44)	8.2×10^{-8}
guaijaverin (45)	1.8×10^{-7}
myrciaphenone A (46)	--------
myrciaphenone B (47)	2.9×10^{-5}
myrciacetin (48)	1.3×10^{-5}
epalrestat	7.2×10^{-8}

The flowers of *Chrysanthemum indicum* L. belongs to compositae family are used for the treatment of eye diseases in Chinese traditional medicine. The inhibitory activity of components isolated from the active fractions of this plant has been examined on RLAR. Among the tested compounds, luteolin **(49)**, luteolin-7-*O*-β-D-glucopyranoside **(50)**, luteolin 7-*O*-β-D-gluopyranosiduronic acid **(51),** acacetin-7-*O*-(6''-α-L-rhamopyranosyl)-β-D-glucopyranoside **(52)** and chlorogenic acid **(53)** showed good inhibition (Table 1.11). But their activity was weaker than that of the commercial synthetic AR inhibitor, eplrestat. In the same experiment the inhibitory effect of the methoxylated flavone, eupatilin **(54),** was much less than the activity of luteolin **(49)** (Yoshikawa *et al.,* 1999).

Table 1.11 Inhibitory activity of compounds from *C. indicum* on RLAR enzyme. (Yoshikawa *et al.,* 1998).

Compounds	IC_{50} at 100µM
luteolin (49),	0.45
luteolin-7-*O*-β-D-glucopyranoside (50)	0.99
luteolin 7-*O*-β-D-gluopyranosiduronic acid(51),	3.1
acacetin-7-*O*-(6''-α-L-rhamopyranosyl)-β-D-glucopyranoside (52)	4.7
and chlorogenic acid (53)	1.8
epalrestat	0.072

Due to the wide biological activities including antioxidative properties reported for green tea, its hot water extract has been examined for AR inhibitory activity. The active fraction purified by solvent fractionation, reversed phase column chromatography, and high performance liquid chromatography gave (+)-catechin **(55)**, (–)-epicatechin **(56)**, (+)-gallocatechin **(57)**, (–)-epigallocatechin **(58)**, (–)-epicatechingallate **(59)** and (–)-epigallocatechingallate **(60)** (Murata *et al.*, 1994). Among these compounds, (–)-epicatechingallate **(59)** (IC_{50} = 38 µmol/L) inhibited AR most strongly, (–)-epicatechin **(56)** (IC_{50} = 79 µmol/L) was next strongest, while (–)-epigallocatechin **(58)** (IC_{50} = 620 µmol/L) did not inhibit the enzyme at all, and (+)-gallocatechin **(57)** inhibited it very weekly (Table 1.12). The results suggested that catechol type catechins inhibited AR more strongly than pyrogallocatechins, and that *epi*-type catechins with a gallolyl group inhibited more strongly than those without. Unlike the inhibitory actions of flavones and flavonols, the inhibitory activity of each catechin appears to be irreversible, because the inhibition was partially restored by adding the enzyme.

Table 1.12 Inhibitory activity of catechins against RLAR enzyme. (Murata *et al.*, 1994).

Compounds	IC_{50} at 100µM
(+)-catechin (55),	280
(–)-epicatechin (56),	79
(+)-gallocatechin (57),	620
(–)-epigallocatechin (58),	>620
(–)-epicatechingallate (59)	38
(–)-epigallocatechingallate (60)	110
Caffeine	480

Sakai *et al.*, (2001) investigated the inhibitory activity of the water extract from commercial English tea against human placenta AR (HPAR). The extract was found to possess a potent activity mainly due to the presence of the flavone glycoside isoquercitrin **(36).** The study also showed that the potency of isoquercitrin **(36)** was equal to that of epalrestat. Enzyme kinetic studies revealed that isoquercitrin **(36)** demonstrated its activity by binding at a site independent of the substrate or cofactor (NADPH) binding sites.

Belamcanda chinensis belongs to iridaceae family, is a perennial shrub growing on the hill sides in the East Asia and have been used as Chinese traditional medicine for the treatment of asthama and tonsillitis. Systematic fractionation of the methanol extract of the rhizomes of *B. chinensis* led to the isolation of 9 isoflavonoids and 3 other phenolic derivatives. All the isolated compounds inhibited AR in RLAR *in vitro* assay. The results summarized in Table 13 indicate that all the compounds possess varying degrees of inhibition (Jung *et al.*, 2002). The isoflavonoids tectoridin (**72**) and tectorigenin (**68**) showed potent activities with IC_{50} values of 1.08 and 1.12 µM, respectively. In the same experiment, the IC_{50} value of tetramethylene glutaric acid was 0.63 µM., the presence of a hydroxyl and a methoxyl group in ring A seem to be essential for the AR inhibitory activity, but the presence of substituents in ring C appeared to have almost no influence on the inhibitory effects. Substitution with methylenedioxy group in ring A markedly reduced the inhibitory activity. As reported by Varma and Kinoshita (1976), inhibition is greater in trihydroxy- than dihydroxyflavones, the hydroxylation at position 4 has beneficial effects, and the abolition of the double bond between C-2 and C-3 leads to a decrease of inhibition. This was shown also to apply for isoflavonoids where trihydroxylated isoflavones such as iristectorene B, tectorigenin and irigenin showed much stronger activity than their dihydroxy counter parts. Furthermore, inhibition was greater in isoflavones with a 4-hydroxyl group.

Table 1.13 Percentage inhibition of isofavonoids and other phenolic compounds isolated from the rhizomes of *Belamcanda chinensis* at a concentration of 10 µM (Jung *et al.*, 2002).

Flavonoid	% Inhibition
Noririsflorentin (**61**)	54.1
Kanzakiflavone-2 (**62**)	60.4
Sheganone (**63**)	37.6
4,7-Di-*O*-Methyltectorigenin (**64**)	45.3
Apocynin (**65**)	33.7
Iristectorene B (**66**)	69.8
p-Hydroxybenzoic acid (**67**)	32.8
Tectorigenin (**68**)	83.5
Irigenin (**69**)	70.9
Irisflorentine (**70**)	40.9
Iridin (**71**)	46.8
Tectoridin (**72**)	83.1

The compositate plant, the flower of *Chrysanthemum indicum* L. has been used for to treat inflammation, fever and eye disease in Chinese traditional preparation. Two flavanone glycosides (2S)- and (2R)-eriodictyol 7-*O*-β-D-glucopyranosiduronic acid (**73** and **74**), and the flavone glycosides apigenin -7-*O*-β-D-glucopyranoside (**75**), diosmetin 7-*O*-β-D-glucopyranoside (**76**) and quercetin 3,7-di-*O*-β-D-glucopyranoside (**77**) isolated from the flowers of *C. indicum* were found to show inhibitory activity on RLAR (Table 14). Among them, **73** and **74** showed potent inhibitory activity (Matsuda *et al.*, 2002a). The methanolic extracts of several natural medicinal food stuffs were shown to possess inhibitory effect on RLAR (Matsuda *et al.,* 2002b). In most cases, bioassay-guided separation resulted in the isolation of flavonoids as active constituents, and among them, quercitrin **(3)**, guaijaverin **(45)** and desmanthin-1 **(44)** exhibited potent inhibitory activity on RLAR. Desmanthin-1 **(44)** (IC_{50} = 0.082 µM) showed the most potent activity, which was equivalent to that of the synthetic ARI, eplrestat (IC_{50} = 0.072 µM). The structural requirements of flavonoids for AR inhibitory activity have been studied by determining the activities of a number of flavonoids and related compounds including flavones, flavonols, flavanones, dihydroflavonol, flavan-3-ols, isoflavones and stilbenes (Matsuda *et al.,* 2002b). The results suggested the following structural requirements:

1. flavones and flavonols having 7-hydroxy and/or catechol moiety (3′ and 4′ dihydroxy group) at the B ring exhibit strong activity;
2. 5-hydroxyl group does not affect activity;
3. 3-hydroxyl and 7-*O*-glucosyl moieties reduce activity;
4. The 2-3 double bond enhances activity; and
5. Flavones and flavonols having the catechol moiety at the B ring exhibit stronger activity than those having the pyrogallol (3′,4′,5′-trihydroxyl) moiety.

Table 1.14 Inhibitiory ativity of compounds isolated from the flowers of *C.indicum* at a concentration of 100 µM (Matsuda *et al.*, 2002a).

Compounds	$IC_{50}(µM)$
(2S)- eriodictyol 7-*O*-β-D-glucopyranosiduronic acid **(73)**	2.1
(2R)-eriodictyol 7-*O*-β-D-glucopyranosiduronic acid **(74)**	1.5
apigenin -7-*O*-β-D-glucopyranoside **(75)**	23
diosmetin 7-*O*-β-D-glucopyranoside **(76)**	23
quercetin 3,7-di-*O*-β-D-glucopyranoside **(77)**	84
epalretat	0.072

Prunus mume belongs to family Rosaceae has been widely cultivated as an ornamental pants, and its fruits is used as a food garnish and drink in Japan. In Chinese traditional medicine, various parts of this plant have been used as herbal medicines. The flowers of *P. mume* have been used for detoxification, expectorant, and sedative purpose and it also used for the treatment of eye disease and skin disorders in Chinese traditional medicine. Yoshikawa *et al.,* (2002) reported the isolation of two previously unknown flavonol oligoglycosides, 2″-*O*-acetylrutin (78) and 2″-*O*-acetyl-3′-*O*-methylrutin **(79),** together with quercetin 3-*O*-(2″,6″-α-L-dirhamnopyranosyl)-β-D-galactopyranoside **(80)**, rutin **(2),** quercetin 3-*O*-neohesperidoside **(81),** and isorhamnetin 3-*O*-rhamnoside **(82)** from the methanolic extract of *Prunus mume,* and determined their inhibitory activity on RLAR. All showed inhibition but the effect of 2"-*O*-acetyl-3'-*O*-methylrutin **(79)** was much higher than the remaining compounds (Table 1.15).

Table 1.15 Inhibitiory ativity of compounds isolated from the flowers of *P. mume* at a concentration of 100 Mm, (Yoshikawa *et al.*, 2002).

Compounds	IC$_{50}$(µM)
2"-*O*-acetylrutin (78) and 2"-*O*-acetyl-3'-*O*-methylrutin **(79)**	9.8
quercetin 3-*O*-(2", 6"-α-L-dirhamnopyranosyl) -β-D-galactopyranoside **(80)**	>30
rutin **(2)**	13
quercetin 3-*O*-neohesperidoside **(81)**	18
isorhamnetin 3-*O*-rhamnoside **(82)**	19
epalretat	0.072

The C-glucosyl flavone, isoaffinetin (83), isolated from the methanolic extract of the dried leaves of *Manilkara indica* showed potent AR inhibitory effect on BLAR, RLAR and HRAR (Haraguchi *et al.*, 2003). Although many ARIs have been reported to inhibit aldehyde reductase, **(83)** failed to show activity against both aldehyde reductase and NADPH oxidase. Like many flavonoidal compounds **(83)** was shown to exert its action by uncompetitive inhibition against both *dl*-glyceraldehyde and NADPH. Structure-activity relationship study revealed that increasing the number of hydroxyl groups in ring B increases inhibition by C-glucosyl flavones.

During a search for possible AR inhibitors from Amazonian plants, the 80% methanol extract of the leaves of *Myrciaria dubia* was found to contain 3 compounds with AR inhibitory activity. The compounds were identified as the phenolic acids: ellagic acid **(84)** and its two derivatives such as 4-*O*-methyl ellagic acid **(85),** 4-(α-rhamnopyranosyl) ellagic acid **(86)** (Ueda *et al.*, 2004).The IC$_{50}$ values of the compounds were 0.27, 0.24, 0.041 and 0.047, 0.14, 0.029 µM in HRAR and RLAR assays, respectively. In HRAR assay, the activity of 4-(α-rhamnopyranosyl) ellagic acid (86) was 60 times more than that of quercetin (IC$_{50}$ = 2.5 µM).

Salacia chinensis is a medicinal plant widely used as antidiabetic in Thailand, Myanmar and India. Phytochemical analysis of the hydroalcoholic extract of the stems of this plant resulted in the isolation of a series of secondary metabolites among which the xanthone, mangiferin **(87)** was one (Morikawa *et al.* 2003). Magniferin (IC$_{50}$ = 3.2 µM) was found to be the most active inhibitor of all the isolated compounds when tested on RLAR. Similarly, the ethyl acetate fraction (IC$_{50}$ = 0.8 ug/mL) of the methanol extract of the fruiting bodies of the bracket fungus *Ganoderma applanatum* showed potent AR inhibitory activity on RLAR

(Lee *et al.*, 2005). Repeated silica gel chromatography yielded several secondary metabolites including the simple phenolic compounds 2,5-dihydroxyacetphenone **(88)**, 2,5-dihydroxybenzoic acid **(89)** and protocatechualdehde **(90)**. Protocatechualdehde **(90)** showed significant inhibitory activity towards RLAR, with an IC_{50} value of 0.7 µg/mL, which is equivalent to that of the positive control tetramethylene glutaric acid (IC_{50} = 0.6 µg/mL). The results suggested that the two phenolic compounds **(89)** and **(90)** having 2,5-dihydroxy benzene moieties exhibit lower AR inhibitory potencies than that carrying a catechol moiety as observed in flavonoids and related compounds.

A number of secondary metabolites have been isolated from the whole plant 80% aqueous acetone extract of *Saussurea medusa* and examined for their inhibitory activity on RLAR (Xie *et al.*, 2005). Among the principal isolated constituents, only the flavonoids and quinic acid derivatives presented in Table 1.16 showed activity.

Table 1.16 Inhibitory effects flavonoids and quinic acid derivatives isolated from the whole plant extract of *Saussurea medusa* Maxim on rat lens aldose reductase (RLAR) (Xie *et al.*, 2005).

Flavonoid	IC_{50} (µM)
Saussuroside A (91)	>100
Saussuroside B (92)	>100
Apigenin (93)	2.2
Apigenin 7-*O*-β-D-glucopyranoside (94)	4.4
Apigenin 4′-*O*-β-D-glucopyranoside (95)	3.2
Apigenin 7-*O*-rutinoside (96)	4.7
Luteolin(49)	0.45
Luteolin 7-*O*-β-D-glucopyranoside (97)	0.99
Luteolin 4′-*O*-β-D-glucopyranoside (98)	4.8
Luteolin 7-O-rutinoside (99)	0.92
Chrysoeriol 7-*O*-β-D-glucopyranoside (100)	26
Chrysoeriol 7-O-rutinoside (101)	14
Quercetin (1)	2.2
Quercetin 3-*O*-β-D-glucopyranoside (102)	4.5
Isorhamnetin 7-*O*-rutinoside (103)	19
3-Caffeoylquinic acid methyl ester (104)	13
4-Caffeoylquinic acid methyl ester (105)	16
5-Caffeoylquinic acid methyl ester (106)	1.3
Eplarestat	0.072

Goodarzi *et al.* (2006) compared the AR inhibitory effects of quercetin **(1)** and naringin **(107)** in streptozotocin-induced diabetic and healthy rats. It was found that AR activity was reduced by 73% and 69% in diabetic rats fed with quercetin (1) and naringin **(107)**, respectively. But, the reduction of enzyme activity in healthy rats was 63% and 59%, respectively. The study revealed that the two flavonoids are effective in reducing of AR activity *in vivo*, particularly in diabetic rats. The seeds of *Aremisia dracunculus*, which have a variety of medicinal uses including as a remedy for diabetes have been investigated for their inhibitory activity on HRAR enzyme. The ethanolic extract of the seeds afforded 4 compounds: 4,5-di-O-caffeoylquinic acid **(108)**, davidigenin **(109)**, 6-demethoxycapillasin **(110)** and 2',4'-dihydroxy-4-methoxydihydrochalcone **(111)**. The compounds displayed either similar or better inhibition than that caused by quercitrin (Logendra *et al.,* 2006). Curcuminoids, curcumin **(112)**, demethoxycurcumin **(113)** and bisdemethoxycurcumin **(114),** isolated from *Curcuma longa* were reported to possess remarkable inhibitory activity on bovine lens AR. It was also observed that curcumin **(112)** exhibited the highest inhibitory activity with IC_{50} value of 6.8 μM (Du *et al.,* 2006). In another study curcumin was shown to delay streptozotocin (STZ)-induced diabetic cataract in rats mainly through its antioxidant property and inhibition of RLAR enzyme (Suryanarayana *et al.,* 2005). Du *et al.* (2006) have also reported that curcuminoids isolated from *Curcuma longa* possess inhibitory activities on BLAR. In the same experiment, the authors synthesized analogues of curcumin and evaluated their ability to inhibit the enzyme. Structure-activity relationship studies revealed that the curcumin analogues with ortho-dihydroxyl groups form a tighter affinity with AR to exert potent activities. In another study curcumin was shown to inhibit bovine kidney AR with an IC_{50} value of 10 μM in a non-competitive manner, but is a poor inhibitor of closely related members of the aldo-keto reductase superfamily, particularly aldehyde reductase (Muthenna *et al.,* 2009)

Similarly, of the stamens of *Nelumbo nucifera* were examined for their possible inhibitory activity on RLAR. Thirteen flavonoids with previously known structures have been isolated from the ethyl acetate soluble fraction of the methanol extract and assessed for their inhibitory activity on RLAR (Lim *et al.,* 2006). The results of the study which are summarized in Table 1.17 indicate that among the isolated compounds, those harboring the 3-*O*-α-L-rhamnopyranosyl-(1→6)-β-D-glucopyranoside group in their C ring, including kaempferol 3-*O*-α-L-rhamnopyranosyl-(1→6)-β-D-glucopyranoside **(119)** (IC_{50} = 5.6 μM) and isorhamnetin 3-*O*-α-L-rhamnopyranosyl-(1→6)-β-D-glucopyranoside **(127)** (IC_{50} = 9.0 μM) possess the highest activity. In addition, arbutin (128) showed weak activity.

Table 1.17 Aldose Reductase (AR) inhibitory activities of flavonoids isolated from the stamens of *Nelumbo nucifera* (Lim *et al.*, 2006).

Flavonoid compound	IC$_{50}$ (µg/ml)	IC$_{50}$ (µM)
Kaemferol (115)	6.94	24
Kaemferol-3-*O*-β-D-galactopyranoside (116)	8.26	18
Kaemferol-7-*O*-β-D-glucopyranoside (117)	6.34	14
Kaemferol-3-*O*-β-D-glucopyranoside (118)	5.05	11
Kaemferol-3-*O*-α-L-rhamnopyranosyl-(1 → 6) β-D-glucopyranoside (119)	3.32	5.6
Kaemferol-3-*O*-α-L-rhamnopyranosyl-(1 → 2) β-D-gluccuronopyranoside (120)	---	
Kaemferol-3-*O*-β-L-rhamnopyranosyl-(1 → 2) β-D-glucopyranoside (121)	---	
Kaemferol-3-*O*-β-D-glucuronopyranoside (122)	-----	
Kaemferol-3-*O*-β-D-glucuronopyranosyl methyl ester (123)	5.52	11.6
Myricetin 3´,5´-dimethyl-3-O-β-D-glucupyranoside (124)	----	
quercetin-3-*O*-β-D-glucuronopyranoside (125)	----	
isorhamnetin -3-*O*-β-D-glucopyranoside (126)	9.13	19
isorhamnetin-3-*O*-α-L-rhamnopyranosyl-(1 → 6) β-D-glucopyranoside (127)	5.86	9.4
Quercetin	5.49	16

In another study involving the leaf extract of *N. nucifera*, it was shown that the ethyl acetate fraction contains quercetin **(1)** and its four of its glycosides: quercetin 3-*O*-β-D-glucopyranoside **(102),** quercetin-3-*O*-β-D-glucuronopyranoside **(125),** quercetin 3-*O*-β-D-galactopyranoside **(129),** and quercetin-3-*O*-β-L-rhamnosyl-(1→6)-β-D-glucopyranoside (rutin) **(2)** as active RLAR inhibitors. Rutin **(2)** (IC$_{50}$ = 2.49 ± 0.04 µM) was the most active of all the isolated flavonoids showing more than twice the activity of quercetin (IC$_{50}$ = 5.54 ± 0.15 µM) (Jung *et al.*, 2008a).

Bioassay-guided fractionation of the MeOH extract of the whole *Viola hondoensis* plant resulted in the isolation of four isoflavonoids, tectoridin-4'-*O*-β-D-glucoside **(130),** tectorigenin **(68),** tectoridin **(72),** and tectorigenin-4'-*O*-β-D-glucoside **(131),** as the active AR inhibitory principles (Moon *et al.*, 2006). Tectoridin-4'-*O*-β-D-glucoside **(130)** (IC$_{50}$ = 0.54 ± 0.02 µM), which contains a glucose moiety at C-7 and C-4' exhibited the most potent inhibitory activity. On the other hand, **(68)** (IC$_{50}$ = 1.12 ± 0.08 µM), which has no substitution at C-7 and C-4' exhibited significantly lower activity than **(130)**. A similar case was observed between compounds **72** and **131**. Tectorigenin-4'-*O*-β-D-glucoside **(131)** without a glucose moiety at C-7 was much more effective than 3, which contains a glucose moiety. These results indicate that glucosylation of C-4′ increases AR inhibitory activity.

In an attempt to obtain nontoxic inhibitors of diabetic complications from edible plants, Kato *et al.* (2006) investigated the hot water extract of the rhizome of *Zingiber officinalis* Roscoe. Out of the 16 phenolic compounds isolated only 5 displayed good inhibitory activity on HRAR. Their structures were identified as (4-hydroxy-3-methoxyphenyl)methanol **(132),** 2-(4-hydroxy-3-methoxyphenyl)ethanol **(133),** 2-(4-hydroxy-3-methoxyphenyl) ethanoic acid **(134),** 2-(-3,4-dimethoxyphenyl) ethanoic acid **(135)** and 4-(4-hydroxy-3-methoxyphenyl)-2-butanone **(136).** Compounds **132, 133,** and **134** exhibited slightly better inhibition than quercetin (IC_{50} = 27.0 ± 3.8 µM), with IC_{50} values of 24.4 ± 4.6, 19.2 ± 1.9 and 18.5 ± 1.1 µM, respectively, whilst the inhibitory potentials of **(135)** and quercetin were almost the same. On the other hand, **(136)** (IC_{50} 197 ± 12 µM) was a much weaker inhibitor than quercetin **(1).** It is interesting to note that [6]-gingerol and [6]-shogaol, the well-known major constituents of ginger displayed extremely weak activities. A structure-activity relationship study revealed that the applicable side alkyl chain length and the presence of a C_3 OCH_3 group in the aromatic ring are essential features for enzyme recognition and binding.

In view of the association between the consumption of pigmented rice and the improvement of human health due to the antioxidant potency of phenolic compounds they contain, the secondary metabolites of black and pigmented brown rice varieties (*Oryza sativa* L. *japonica*) have been investigated (Yawadio *et al.*, 2006). Two anthocyanins: cyanidin-3-*O*-β-glucoside **(137)** and peonidin-3-*O*-β-glucoside **(138)** were isolated from black rice, whilst the major component of pigmented brown rice was found to be ferulic acid **(139).** All the isolated compounds showed inhibitory activity on BLAR with compound **(138)** (IC_{50} = 8.7 µg/mL) exhibiting the highest activity that was better than that of quercetin (IC_{50} = 11.4 µg/mL). It was concluded that black and brown pigmented rice varieties possess marked health benefits in preventing diabetic complications by preventing the key enzyme (AR) involved in their development.

Origanum vulgare ssp. hirtum traditionally used in Morocco for the control and treatment of diabetes, was studied for its inhibitory activity against RLAR (Koukoulitsa *et al.,* 2006). The polar extracts of the plant growing wild in Greece yielded 3 phenolic acids: caffeic acid **(140),** rosmarinic acid and **(141),** lithospermic acid B **(142)** along with 2 terpenoidal compounds. The inhibitory activity against RLAR of compounds **140–142** was examined and docking studies on the active site of the enzyme were performed. The most active compound was found to be lithospermic acid B **(142)** inhibiting the enzyme by 96% at a dose of 100 µM. Caffeic acid **(140)** was inactive. Docking results seem to support the biological data. Despite the fact that carboxylic acids have a potent inhibitory activity *in vitro*, they were less potent *in vivo* due to their complete dissociation at physiological pH.

Black bamboo, *Phyllostachys nigra* grows particularly in Southeast Asia and is widely used as a source of food. The leaves of *P. nigra* were investigated for their inhibitory effect on rat lens ALR2 to evaluate their potential for treatment of diabetic complications. The investigation led to the isolation and identification of the flavones isoorientin **(143)**, orientin **(144)**, vitexin **(145)** luteolin 6-*C*-(6″-*O*-*trans*-caffeoyl glucoside) **(146)**, vittariflavone **(147)** and tricin **(148)**), and the simple phenolic acids, *cis*-coumaric acid **(149)**, and *p*-coumaric acid **(150)** that inhibited ALR2 activity (Jung *et al.*, 2007). Of these, luteolin 6-*C*-(6″-*O*-*trans*-caffeoylglucoside) **(146)** (IC$_{50}$ = 0.0134 µM) was found to exhibit the strongest inhibition. In the same experiment, the inhibitory potency of reference compound tetramethyl glutaric acid (IC$_{50}$ = 0.924 µM) was much lower.

Finger millet, *Eleusine coracana* is a good source of polyphenols among cereals. Finger millet polyphenols being a major antidiabetic and antioxidant components, Chethan *et al.*, (2008) evaluated their AR inhibiting activity. It was shown that the phenolic constituents in finger millet such as gallic acid **(151)**, protocatechuic acid **(152)**, *p*-hydroxy benzoic acid **(153)**, *p*-coumaric acid **(150)**, vanillic acid **(154)**, syringic acid **(155)**, ferulic acid **(139**), *trans*-cinnamic acid **(156)** and the quercetin **(1)** inhibited cataract eye lens effectively, the latter was more potent with an IC$_{50}$ of 14.8 nM. Structure relationship analysis revealed that OH group at position 4 was important for AR inhibitory property. It was also observed that the presence of O-methyl group next to the carbon carrying the phenolic OH moiety eliminates AR activity. The phenolic acids were found to inhibit AR reversibly by non-competitive inhibition.

The methanol extract of the air-dried fruit pericarp of the tropical and subtropical edible fruit, Litchi (*Litchi chinensis Sonn.*) was investigated for its inhibitory activity on RLAR. The ethyl acetate soluble fraction of the methanol extract afforded four compounds of which 2,5-dihydroxybenzoic acid **(89)**, delphinidin 3-*O*-β-galactopyranoside-3′,5′-di-*O*-β-glucopyranoside **(157)**, and delphinidin 3-*O*-β- galactopyranoside-3′-*O*-β-glucopyranoside **(158)** showed inhibitory activity on RLAR assay (Lee *et al.*, 2009). However, the anthocyanin delphinidin 3-*O*-β-galactopyranoside-3′-*O*-β-glucopyranoside **(158)** exhibited the most powerful activity with an IC$_{50}$ value of 0.23 µg/mL, which was twice that of the positive control tetramethylene glutaric acid (IC$_{50}$ = 0.48 µg/mL).

Phytochemical analysis of the 80% methanolic extract of the roots of *Pueraria thunbergiana* led to the isolation of four isoflavonoids; daidzein **(159)**, daidzin **(160)**, puerarin **(161)** and ononin **(162)**, and all showed inhibitory activity against RLAR. In addition, the isoflavonoids: genistin **(163)**, genistein **(164)**, and formononetin **(165)**, and the flavonoids baicalin **(166)**, baicalein **(167)**, were examined and showed inhibitory activity against RLAR (Park *et al.*, 2007). Structure-activity relationship among these compounds revealed that the aglycones possess better inhibition than the corresponding glycosides and substitution of the C-4' OH group with a methoxyl group reduce activity. Engeletin **(168)** and astilbin **(169)**, dihydro flavonol glycosides isolated from the ethyl acetate extract of the leaves of *Stelechocarpus cauliflorus* R.E. Fr. were found to possess AR inhibitory activity. Although engeletin **(168)** has only one hydroxyl group in its C ring as opposed to astilbin **(39)**, which contains two hydroxyl groups at 3' and 4' positions, the inhibitory activity of the former against HRAR was 23 times greater than that the latter and twice that of quercetin **(1)** (Wirasathien *et al.*, 2007).

Viola hondoensis belongs to family Violaceae is distributed in the southern part of Korea. In traditional medicine, the herb has been used as an expectorant and a treatment for skin eruption. The isolation and characterization of ARIs from the *V. hondoensis* W. Becker et H Boss has been reported (Chung *et al.*, 2008). The MeOH extract (IC_{50} = 1.2 µg/mL) and EtOAc fraction (0.6 µg/mL) were found to exhibit potent RLAR inhibition *in vitro* (Table 1.18). Kakkalide **(169)** (IC_{50} = 0.3 µg/mL), the major isoflavonoid glycoside isolated from the ethyl acetate soluble fraction was found to be more the active constituent of the plant, which is compared with positive control TMG (tetramethylene glutaric acid).

Table 1.18 Inhibitory Effects of the Extract, Solvent Fractions and Compound of *Viola hondoensis* on Rat Lens Aldose Reductase. (Chung *et al.*, 2008).

Fractions and Compounds	IC_{50}(µg/mL)
MeOH extract	1.28
n-Hexane fraction	6.2
EtOAc fraction	0.62
Chloroform fraction	3.2
n-BuOH fraction	4.3
Kakkalide	0.34
TMG (tetramethylene glutaric acid)	0.48

Rhus verniciflua grows particularly in South East Asia and the biological activities of this plant have been reported as anti-inflammatory, anti-cancer, and anti-rheumatoid arthritis *etc*. In an attempt to find to find potential AR inhibitors, Lee *et al.* 2008 investigated the ethanol extract of the bark of *Rhus verniciflua*, a plant that grows particularly in South East Asia and the pharmacological activities of this plant have been reported as anti-inflammatory, anti-cancer, and anti-rheumatoid arthritis *etc*. Several compounds including flavanonols, flavones, an aurone, a chalcone and simple phenolics have been isolated from the active ethyl acetate fraction (IC$_{50}$ = 0.6 µg/mL), which showed concentration dependent inhibition. The isolated compounds were identified as fustin **(170)**, morin hydrate **(171)**, fisetin **(172)**, quercetin **(1)**, sulfuretin **(173)**, butein **(174)**, protocatechuic acid **(152)**, and ethyl gallate **(175)**. The chalcone butein **(174)** exhibited the strongest inhibitory activity against HRAR with an IC$_{50}$ value of 0.7 µM, a better inhibition than that displayed by epalrestat (Table 1.19). The activity of sulfuretin **(173)** with aurone structure also showed inhibition that was equal to the reference drug epalrestat.

Table 1.19 Inhibitory Effects of the Compounds Isolated from the Bark of *R. verniciflua* on RHALR2 (Lee *et al.* 2008)

Compounds	Conc. (µm)	%inhibition	IC$_{50}$ (µM)
Epalrestat	2.5	85.8±5.0	1.3
	1.25	49.1±1.7	
	0.625	11.8±4.2	
fustin (170),	2	20.1±0.5	>2
morin hydrate (171)	2	14.1±8.0	>2
fisetin (172),	2	31.1_8.9	>2
quercetin (1),	2	39.1±4.6	>2
sulfuretin (173	2.0	69.8_3.3	1.3
	1.0	41.9±1.1	
	0.5	7.0_2.3	
butein (174)	2.0	89.9±7.7	0.7
	1.0	65.1_1.1	
	0.5	41.1_2.2	
protocatechuic acid (152),	2	12.6±3.7	>2
ethyl gallate (175).	2.0	----	>2
pentagalloyl glucose	2.0	46.6_5.1	>2

Sorbus domestica fruits (Rosaceae) are widely used in northern Europe as antioxidant agents in beverages. The diethyl ether and ethyl acetate extracts of *S. domestica* fruits possess AR inhibitory activity. Further analysis of these extracts revealed that the AR inhibitory activity is attributed to the high flavonoids and hydroxyl cinnamoyl content of the plant (Termentzi *et al.*, 2008).

From the methanolic extract of the dried whole plant of *Sinocrassula indica* (Crassulaceae) thirty-one flavonoids were isolated. Among the isolated flavonoid constituents, the inhibitory effects of eight principal components were investigated on RLAR enzyme (Morikawa *et al.* 2008). It was found that luteolin **(49)**, quercetin **(1)**, multiflorin B **(176)**, quercetin 3-O-β-D-glucopyranoside **(102)**, kaempferol **(115)**, sinocrassosides A_2 **(177)**, sinocrassosides D_2 **(178)**, and quercetin-3-O-β-D-glucopyranosyl-7-O-α-L-rhamnopyranoside **(179)**, have activities with IC_{50} values shown in Table 1.20.

Table 1.20 Inhibitory Effects of the Compounds Isolated from the whole plant of *Sinocrassula indica* on RLAR. (Morikawa *et al.* 2008).

Compounds	$IC_{50}(\mu M)$
kaempferol **(115)**	10.0
quercetin **(1)**	2.2
quercetin 3-O-β -D-glucopyranoside **(102)**	4.5
sinocrassosides D2**(178)**	47
sinocrassosides A2**(177)**	31
multiflorin B **(176)**	2.7
quercetin 3-O-β -D-glucopyranosyl-7-O-α -L-rhamnopyranoside **(179)**	56
luteolin **(49)**	0.45
multiflorin B **(176),**	2.2

Cirsium maackii, a member of the Asteraceae family, is a perennial thistle that grows abundantly in Korea. The whole plants of Cirsium species (Cirsii Radix et Herba) have been used as a folk medicine in the treatment of hemorrhaging, inflammation of the liver and kidney, and a variety of abdominal and intestinal disorders. Jung *et al.* (2009) have assessed the AR inhibitory activity of the leaves, roots, stems, and flowers of the Korean thistle, *C. maackii* along with two major components, luteolin 5-O-β-D-glucopyranoside **(180)** and the aglycone luteolin **(49)** against RLAR and HRAR (Table 1.21). HPLC quantitative analysis of the two key flavonoids in each plant parts indicated that the content of **180** and **49** might contribute to the antioxidant and AR inhibitory activities of *C. maackii*.

Table 1.21 AR Inhibitiory ativity of isolated compounds from *Cirsium maackii*, (Jung *et al.* 2009).

Compounds	IC_{50} (μM)	
	RLAR	**HRAR**
luteolin 5-O-β-D-glucopyranoside (180)	0.33 ± 0.00	6.07 ± 0.05
luteolin (49)	0.52 ± 0.05	9.18 ± 0.10
Quercetin	1.53 ± 0.20	14.79 ± 0.35
Epalrestat	0.07 ± 0.00	0.07 ± 0.01

Sophora flavescens Ait belongs to family Leguminosceae is a perennial shrub that occurs in the wild and is also cultivated throughout North East Asia. The dried root of *S. flavescens*, Sophorae Radix, is an important herbal medicine that is used in folk medicine as an antipyretic, analgesic, anthelmintic and stomachic, and is used for the treatment of gastrointestinal haemorrhage, diarrhoea and eczema. The root extracts of *Sophora flavescens* and its prenylated flavonoids, which are known to exhibit antidiabetic activities in several enzymatic systems (Kim *et al.*, 2006) and inhibit the Na^+-glucose cotransporter (Sato *et al.*, 2007) implicated in diabetes have been examined for their AR inhibitory activities (Jung *et al.*, 2008b). The results summarized in Table 22 indicated that all of the prenylated flavonoids isolated from the active methylene dichloride and ethyl acetate fractions show varying degrees of activity on both RLAR and HRAR assays. The inhibitory effect of the prenylated chalcone desmethylanhydroicaritin **(181)** (IC_{50} = 0.95 ± 0.04 µM), however, was the highest on RLAR assay. In this assay, the IC_{50} values of epalrestat and quercetin were 0.28 ± 0.01 and 7.73 ± 0.29 µM, respectively. Similarly, in the HRAR assay most of the compounds showed marked inhibitory activity with the prenylated flavanone (2S)-7,4'-dihydroxy-5-methoxy-8-(γ,γdimethylally)-flavanone **(192)** (IC_{50} = 0.37 µM) exerting the highest activity, which was better than quercetin (IC_{50} = 2.54 µM) and comparable with that of epalrestat (IC_{50} = 0.28 µM). Overall, the prenylated flavanones and prenylated flavonols showed higher activities than the prenylated chalcones in the RLAR assay, whereas the prenylated chalcones and the prenylated flavonols exhibited greater activity than the prenylated flavanones in the HRAR assay.

Table 1.22 IC_{50} Inhibitory activities values of prenylated flavonoids isolated from the root extract of *Sophora flavescens* against rat lens aldose reuctase (RLAR) and human recombinant aldose eductase (HRAR) (Jung *et al.*, 2008b).

Flavonoid	RLAR		HRAR	
	µgmL^{-1}	µM	µgmL^{-1}	µM
Desmethylanhydroicartin (181)	0.34	0.95	0.16	0.45
8-Lavandulylkaempferol (182)	1.61	3.80	0.33	0.79
Kushenol C (183)	8.12	18.54	0.37	0.85
Kuraridinol (184)	10.10	22.14	0.60	1.32
Kuraridin (185)	9.46	21.60	0.12	0.27
Xanthohumol (186)	3.80	10.73	-----	----
Sophoraflavanone (187)	25.26	59.58	0.60	1.42
Kurarinol (188)	0.97	2.13	2.0	4.39
Kurarinone (189)	1.31	2.99	1.67	3.81
(2S)-2'-Methoxykurarinone (190)	1.70	3.77	5.0	11.0

Table 1.22 *Contd...*

Flavonoid	RLAR		HRAR	
	μgmL^{-1}	μM	μgmL^{-1}	μM
(2S)-3β,7,4′-Trihydroxy-5-methoxy-8-(γ,γ-dimethylallyl)-flavanone (191)	1.34	3.63	1.67	4.50
(2S)-7,4′-Dihydroxy-5-methoxy-8-(γ,γ-dimethylallyl)-flavanone (192)	11.57	32.69	0.13	0.37
Kushenol E (193)	3.29	7.74	0.89	2.09
Leachianone (194)	4.62	12.97	0.89	2.49
Quercetin	2.61	7.73	0.86	2.54
Epalrestat	0.09	0.28	0.09	0.28

The roots and rhizomes of licorice species (*Glycyrrhiza* sp.) have for long been used, worldwide, as herbal medicine and natural sweetener. Licorice is also known to improve glucose tolerance in diabetic mice. Such preventive and inhibitory activities against diabetes, shown by several licorice-derived components led to further investigation of the inhibitory effects of *Glycyrrhiza uralensis* on diabetic complications. The investigation which involved extraction of the dried rhizomes of the plant with methylene chloride resulted in the isolation of 5 prenylated flavonoids: semilicoisoflavone B **(195)**, 7-*O*-methylluteone **(196)**, dehydroglyasperin C **(197)**, dehydroglyasperin D **(198)**, and isoangustone A **(199)**, and three non-prenylated flavonoids: liquiritigenin **(200)**, isoliquiritigenin **(201)**, and licochalcone A **(202)**, among others. Semilicoisoflavone B **(195)** was the most potent inhibitor with IC_{50} values of 1.8 and 10.6 μM against RLAR and HRAR, respectively. The IC_{50} values of epalrestat in the two assays were shown in table 1.23. In the kinetic analyses using Lineweaver–Burk plots of 1/velocity and 1/concentration of substrate, semilicoisoflavone B **(195)** showed noncompetitive inhibition against RLAR. The results of the study indicated that the presence of a γ,γ-dimethylchromene ring is partly responsible for the AR inhibitory activity of isoprenoid-type flavonoids (Lee *et al* 2010).

Table 1.23 Inhibitory Effects of the Compounds Isolated from *Glycyrrhizae uralensis* on Rat Lens AR and Recombinant Human AR. (Lee *et al* 2010).

Compounds	IC_{50} (μM)	
	RLAR	HRAR
Quercetin	2.5	12.7
Epalrestat	0.9	1.0
semilicoisoflavone B (195),	1.8	10.6
7-*O*-methylluteone (196),	28.5	76.5
dehydroglyasperinC (197),	42.7	130.6
dehydroglyasperin D (198),	62.4	176.2
and isoangustone A (199),	99.5	280.8
liquiritigenin (200)	2.0	21.9
isoliquiritigenin (201)	3.4	27.5
licochalcone A (202)	96.3	257.2

Lee *et al.* 2011 reported the isolation of the flavanol glycoside, glucodistylin (**203**) and three polyphenol derivatives: gallate (**204**), (+)-catechin (**55**) and (+)-gallocatechin (**57**) from an aqueous acetone extract of the bark of *Quercus acutissima*. The most active compound glucodistylin exhibited uncompetitive inhibitory activity against RHAR with an IC_{50} value of 7.2 µM, activity that was twice that of quercetin (Table 1.24).

Table 1.24 Inhibitory effects of compounds isolated from *Q. acutissima* on HRAR. (Lee *et al.* 2011).

Compounds	$IC_{50}(µM)$
quercetin	15.98
glucodistylin (**203**)	7.2
gallate (**204**),	------
(+)-catechin (**55**)	112.5>
(+)-gallocatechin (**57**)	159.4>

The young leaves of *Artemisia montana* (Nakai) Pampan are consumed as foodstuffs, and the mature plant used as a moxibustion in Korea and Japan. Bioassay-guided fractionation of extract of the whole plant yielded RLAR inhibitory active ethyl acetate and n-butanol fractions. Repeated column chromatography of the fractions afforded a series of chlorogenic acids and flavonoids, among others (Jung *et al.*, 2011). The isolated acids: 3,5-di-*O*-caffeoylquinic acid (**205**), chlorogenic acid (**53**), cryptochlorogenic acid (**206**) and neochlorogenic acid (**207**) inhibited RLAR with IC_{50} values shown in table 1.25. The flavonoids obtained: apigenin (**93**), luteolin (**49**), quercetin (**1**), isoquercitrin (**36**), hyperoside (**208**), luteolin 7-rutinoside(scolymoside)(**99**) displayed better activity than the plant acids with (**49**) (IC_{50} = 0.19 ± 0.02) exhibiting the most potent effect followe by (**1**) (IC_{50} = 0..30 ± 0.03) and (**99**) (IC_{50} = 0.55 ± 0.03).

Table 1.25 Inhibitory effects of compounds isolated from *A. montana* on RLAR. (Jung *et al.*, 2011).

Compounds	$IC_{50}(µM)$
3,5-di-*O*-caffeoylquinic acid (**205**),	5.37±0.25
chlorogenic acid (**53**),	4.36±0.47
cryptochlorogenic acid (**206**)	11.13±1.70
neochlorogenic acid (**207**)	19.19±2.19
apigenin (**93**),	0.67±0.03
luteolin (**49**),	0.19±0.02
quercetin (**1**),	0.30±0.03
isoquercitrin (**36**),	1.16±0.0
hyperoside (**208**),	1.85±0.06
luteolin 7-rutinoside(scolymoside) (**99**)	0.55±0.03
Umbeliferone (259)	122.10±12.26
Scoparone (260)	44.30±0.47
Scopoletin (251)	64.50±9.08
Esculetin (261)	172.48±9.01
Scopolin (262)	128.15±1.72

Chlorogenic acid (1), 3,5-di-O-caffeoylquinic acid (2), apigenin (3), 1,3, 5-tri-O-caffeoylquinic acid (4), 5,7-dimethoxy-flavanone-40-O-[-Dapiofuranosyl-(12)]-D-glucopyranoside (5), and b-sitosterol (6) from 70% methanolic leaves extact of *Phoradendron* sp. the IC_{50}s of compounds 1, 2, and 4 toward AR were 6.83 lM, 4.62 lM, and 4.28 lM, while compounds 3, 5, and 6 were inactive (Zhiqiang *et al.*, 2017).

Effects of 95% ethanol extracts from the leaves of *C. esculenta* and, its organic solvent soluble fractions, including the dichloromethane (CH_2Cl_2), ethyl acetate (EtOAc), *n*-butanol (BuOH) and water (H_2O) layers, using DL-glyceraldehyde as a substrate. Ten compounds, namely tryptophan (**1**), orientin (**2**), isoorientin (**3**), vitexin (**4**), isovitexin (**5**), luteolin-7-*O*-glucoside (**6**), luteolin-7-*O*-rutinoside (**7**), rosmarinic acid (**8**), 1-*O*-feruloyl-D-glucoside (**9**) and 1-*O*-caffeoyl-D-glucoside (**10**) were isolated from the EtOAc and BuOH fractions of *C. esculenta*. All the isolates were subjected to an *in vitro* bioassay to evaluate their inhibitory activity against rat lens aldose reductase. Among tested compounds, compounds **2** and **3** significantly inhibited rat lens aldose reductase, with IC_{50} values of 1.65 and 1.92 μM, respectively. Notably, the inhibitory activity of orientin was 3.9 times greater than that of the positive control, quercetin (4.12 μM) (Hong *et al.*, 2014).

Terpenoids

Terpenoids are the most numerous and structurally diverse family of natural products derived from C_5 isoprene units. For many years, pharmaceutical and food industries have exploited them for their potentials as effective medicines and flavor enhancers. Considering the numbers and diversity of this group of secondary metabolites, however, literature reports on their AR inhibitory activity is not numerous.

Moon *et al.*, 1988 started research on monoterpine derivate to find BLAR enzyme Inhibitory activity. Most of the monoterpine showed the mild inhibitory activity on BLAR. Only 3-carene showed no effect on the enzyme activity at the concentration of 10^{-3}M (Table 1.26). Among them, (+) Pulegon showed maximum activity with 42% inhibition at the 10^{-3}M concentration.

Fujita *et al.*, 1995 reported that the monoterpene glycosides: perillosides A (**209**), B (**210**), C (**211**) and D (**212**) isolated from the leaves of *Perilla frutescens* possess potent inhibitory activity on both RLAR and HRAR enzymes. But, the inhibitory effects of perillosideB (**210**) and perilloside D (**212**) were much lower than perilloside A (**210**) and perilloside C (**211**) though their structures are similar to those of **209** and **211.** Structure-activity relationship among this group of compounds was carried out by synthesizing several related monoterpene glycosides and their tetraactates and determining the AR inhibitory effects. It was concluded that a planner monoterpene glucoside consisting of a *p*-menthane skeleton with an equatorial side chain and a β-D-glucosyloxy moiety at the C-7 position is expected to have a potent inhibitory effect on AR enzymes. Kinetic studies revealed that the type of inhibition by perilloside A (**209**) and perilloside C (**211**) was competitive with respect glyceraldehydes, whilst the inhibition caused by their tetraacetates was non-competitive.

Table 1.26 RLAR Inhibitiory ativity of some monoterpines
(Moon *et al.*, 1988).

Compounds	%inhibition (M)	
	10^{-3}	10^{-5}
3-Carene	0	0
4-Caranol	23	17
4-Isocaranon	21	14
3-Hydroxy methyl- caran-4-on	22	17
3-Hydroxy methyl- caran-4-ol	30	16
(+)Carvon	25	14
(-)Carvon	35	14
Carbomethon	37	21
(+)Pulegon	42	20
(-)isopulegol	25	17
(-)Menthon	23	05
4-Hydroxy methyl- Menthon	31	17
Camphor	14	05

The abietane-type diterpenoids: danshenols A (**213**) and B (**214**), dihydrotanshinone I (**215**), tanshinone I (**26**), cryptotanshinone (**217**), tanshinone II A (**218**) and (-)-danshexinkun A (**219**) isolated from the dried root and rhizome of *Salvia miltiorhiza* showed inhibitory activity against RLAR enzyme. Among these danshenol A (**213**) was found to exhibit the most potent inhibitory activity with an IC_{50} value of 0.10 µg/mL. In the same experiment, the IC_{50} value of the reference drug epealrestat was 0.10 µg/mL (Kasimu *et al.*, 1997). Yoshikawa *et al.* 1999, isolated 6 sesquiterpenes from the methanol extract of the dried flowers of *Chrysanthemum indicum*, which showed inhibitory activity on RLAR. However, the tested compounds: clovanediol (**220**), caryolane 1,9-β-diol (**221**), oplopanone (**222**), kikkanol A (**223**) and kikkanol C (**224**) showed weak inhibitory activity, indicating that the sesquiterpenes do not contribute to much of the AR activity of the plant.

The hydroalcoholic extract of the stems of *Salacia chinensis* afforded a series of triterpenes and one sesqiterpene. However, only two of the isolated oleanane-type triterpenes, 3β,22β-dihydroxyolean-12-en-29-oic acid (225) (IC_{50} = 26.0 µM) and maytenfolic acid (226) (IC_{50} = 72.0 µM), and all of the norfriedelane-type triterpenes, tingenone (227) (IC_{50} = 13.0

µM), tingenin B (228) (IC_{50} = 7.0 µM) and regeol A (IC_{50} = 30.0 µM) (229) and triptocalline A (230) (IC_{50} = 14 µM) showed activity on RLAR. The friedelane- and ursane- type triterpenes as well as the eudesmane-type sesquiterpene failed to exhibit appreciable activity (Morikawa *et al.*, 2003). Similarly, investigation of the hydroalcoholic root extracts of another *Salacia* species, *S. oblonga* used in Ayurvedic traditional medicine in India as a remedy for diabetes among others, were investigated for their inhibitory activity against RLAR. The principal components of the active ethyl acetate soluble fraction yielded diterpenes and tritepenes. The triterpenes obtained were kotalagenin 16-acetate (231), maytenfolic acid (226), 3β, 22-α-dihydroxyolean-12-en-29-oic acid (225) and 26-hydroxy-1,3-friedalnedione (232), 19-hydroxyferruginol (233) and lambertic acid (234) were the diterpene constituents of the plant. Among the isolated compounds, 3β, 22-α-dihydroxyolean-12-en-29-oic acid (225) was the most active exerting a percentage inhibition of 75.9% at a concentration of 100 µM (Matsuda *et al.*, 1999). Similarly, 12-hydroxyjasmonic acid 12-*O*-β-glucopyranoside (235), and *p*-menth-3-ene-1, 2-diol-1-*O*-β-glucopyranoside (236) isolated from the polar extract of *Origanum vulgare* showed AR inhibitory activity. At a concentration of 100 µg/mL the compounds showed percent inhibition of 77 ± 1.4 and 41 ± 0.6, respectively (Koukoulitsa *et al.*, 2006).

Fatmawati *et al.* 2010a isolated ganoderic acid Df (237), a lanostane-type triterpenoid from the fruiting body of *Ganoderma lucidum* Df. Ganoderic acid Df (237), showed potent inhibitory activity against HRAR with an IC_{50} value of 22.8 µM. The carboxyl group in the side chain of (237) was found to be essential for eliciting inhibitory activity as its methyl ester derivative was much less active.

In another study, the chloroform extract of the fruiting body of *G. lucidum* was found to show inhibitory activity on HRAR *in vitro*. From the acidic fraction, two potent human ARIs, ganoderic acid C2 (**238**) and ganoderenic acid A (**239**), were isolated together with three related compounds (Fatmawati *et al.* 2010b). The free carboxyl group of (**238**) and (**239**) was considered to be essential in eliciting the inhibitory activity. The COOH hydrophilic head of (**238**) and (**239**) is similar to that of many ARIs such as tolrestat and zopolrestat, and this head can possibly bind to AR in the form $(COO)^-$.

Alkaloids

Although alkaloids are by far the most biologically active secondary metabolites, there appear to have been very few reports in the literature concerning their AR inhibition effect. One such report by Kubo *et al.* (1994) deals with the isolation of 7 alkaloidal components dehydrocorydaline (**240**) from the methanolic extract of the tuber of

Corydalis turtschaninovii. Among these alkaloids only the quaternary alkaloidal component, dehydrocorydaline (**240**) produced inhibition against RLAR. All the tertiary alkaloids failed to show activity. Similarly, Lee, 2002b characterized the isoquinoline alkaloids, berberine chloride (**241**) and palmatine iodide (**242**) as AR inhibitors of methanol extract of the root of *Coptis japonica*. The IC_{50} values of the alkaloids against RLAR were found to be 13.98 and 13.45 μM. In the same experiment the isoquinoline alkaloids, berberine sulfate (**243**) berberine iodide (**244**) and palmatine sulfate (**245**) were also tested. It was observed that inhibitory activities of the chlorinated and sulfated analogues are much greater than those for the iodide (Lee, 2002b).

In the search for components inhibiting AR, Kato *et al.* (2009) isolated an active alkaloid from the hot water extract of *Evodia rutaecarpa* Bentham. The alkaloid identified as N2-(2-methyl amino benzoyl) tetrahydro-1H-pyrido[3,4-b] indol-1-one (rhetsinine) (**246**) inhibited HRAR with an IC_{50} value of 24.1 μM.

Coumarins

The coumarin (benzopyran-2-one, or chromen-2-one) ring system, present in natural products (such as the anticoagulant warfarin) displays interesting pharmacological properties. The AR inhibitory activities of 41 coumarins have been included in the review by Kawannishi et al. (2003). The hot water root extract of *Angelica gigas* has been reported to inhibit BLAR at a concentration of 100 μg/mL. Three linear coumarins: decursunol angelate (**247**), decursin (**248**) and nodakenin (**249**) with AR inhibitory activity have been isolated. Among these, nodakenin (**249**) exhibited significant inhibition with an IC_{50} value of 7.33 μM (Lee *et al.*, 2002). Other workers have reported the isolation of 11 coumpounds, 9 of which were coumarins, from the dried stem of *A. gigas* with AR inhibitory activity. Isoimperatorin (**250**), scopoletin (**251**), and 3'-hydroxyxanthyletin (**252**) showed good inhibitory activity with IC_{50} values of 5.1, 2.59, and 4.23 μM, respectively. 7-Methoxy-5-prenyloxycoumarin (**253**), bergapten (**254**) and psoralen (**255**) also showed an intermediate activity with IC_{50} values of 32.38, 25.03, and 51.62 μM, respectively. Xanthotoxin (256) ($IC_{50} = 103.15$ μM) showed weak activity. Imperatorin (**257**) and decursin (**248**) did not show any significant activity. Interestingly, visaminol (**258**), which is not a coumarin but a chromone derivative, showed relatively good inhibitory activity with an IC_{50} value of 26.66 μM (Park *et al.*2011).

In another study, five coumarins: umbelliferone (**259**), scoparone (**260**), scopoletin (**251**), esculetin (**261**), and scopolin (**262**) with AR inhibitory activity were isolated from the whole plant extract of *Artemisia montana*. All the other isolated compounds showed intermediate activities but the inhibition produced by scoparone (**260**) (IC$_{50}$ = 44.30 ± 0.47 μM) on RLAR was better than the others (Jung *et al.*, 2011).

Tannins

Tannins have diverse effects on the biological systems because they are potential metal ion chelators, protein precipitating agents and biological antioxidants. Lee *et al.*, 2008. Isolated the one tannin pentagalloyl glucose (**263**) from the *Rhus verniciflua*, it shows the inhibitory activity against AR.

Miscellaneous

Two polyacylated sucroses prunose I (**264**) and prunose II (**265**) were isolated from the methanolic extract of *Prunus mume*. Whilst (**264**) (IC$_{50}$ = 58 μM) exhibited inhibitory effect against RLAR, the effect of (**265**) (IC$_{50}$ = >100 μM) was very weak (Yoshikawa *et al.,* 2002) The bark of *Cinnammum cassia*, the commercial source of cinnamon, was subjected to methanol extraction and fractionated with various solvents. Further investigation of the active hexane fraction led to the isolation of *trans*-cinnamaldehyde (**266**), cinnamyl alcohol (**267**) and eugenol (**268**), among others. (**266**) (IC$_{50}$ = 3 μg/mL) exhibited good inhibitory activity, whereas the activities of (**267**) and (**268**) (IC$_{50}$ = 500 μg/mL) was much weaker (Lee 2002a). Cerebrosides (**269**) (30.0 The μg/mL) isolated from the EtOAc soluble fraction of the methanol extract of the fruiting bodies of *Ganoderma applanatum* showed inhibition against RLAR (Lee *et al.*, 2005). The essential oil obtained from the seeds of *Cuminum cyminum* was found to completely inhibit RLAR at a dose of 0.5 mg/mL. Chromatographic analysis of the oil by HPLC reveled that cuminaldehyde (**270**) is the active constituent of the oil. Cuminaldehyde (**270**) (IC$_{50}$ = 0.80 μM) displayed a potent activity that could be compared with the reference compound quercetin (IC$_{50}$ = 0.51 μM) (Lee, 2005).

Conclusion

Prevention of diabetic complications has become the current interest of scientists and research workers worldwide. Use of plant derived phytochemicals in the treatment of various chronic disorders is increasing and many phytomedicines are becoming the best alternatives to synthetic drugs. Diabetic and its complications can be prevented using phytomedicines. The promising plant derived compounds like quercetin (**1**), kaempferol (**115**), and ellagic acid (**84**) have long standing evidences for their AR inhibitory activity. In the present context this review stresses the need to focus on research for potential phytochemical compounds which can be effectively used for the treatment of diabetic complications.

References

Angel de la Fuente J, Manzanaro S. 2003. Aldose reductase inhibitors from natural sources. Nat Prod Rep 20: 243–251.

Brownlee M. 2001. Biochemistry and molecular cell biology of diabetic complications. Nature 414: 813-820.

Cerelli MJ, Curtis DL, Dunn JP et al.1986. Antiinflammatory and aldose reductase inhibitory activity of some tricyclic arylacetic acids. J Med Chem 29: 2347–2351

Chethan S, Dharmesh SM, Malleshi NG et al. 2008. Inhibition of aldose reductase from cataracted eye lenses by finger millet (Eleusine coracana) polyphenols. Bioorg Med Chem 16: 10085-10090.

Chung IM, Kim MY, Park WH et al. 2008. Aldose reductase inhibitors from Viola hondoensis. Am J Chin Med 36: 799-803.

Chung YS, Choi YH, Lee SJ et al. 2005. Water extract of Aralia elata prevents cataractogenesis in vitro and in vivo. J Ethanopharmacol 101: 49-54.

Costantino L, Rastelli G, Vianello P et al. 1999. Diabetes complications and their potential prevention: Aldose reductase inhibition and other approaches. Med Res Rev 19: 3-23.

Crabbe MJ, Goode D. 1998. Aldose reductase: a window to the treatment of diabetic complication?. Prog Retin Eye Res 17: 313-383.

Du ZY, Bio YD, Liu Z et al. 2006. Curcumin analogs as potent aldose reductase inhibitors. Arch Pharm 339: 123-128.

Fatmawati S, Kurashiki K, Takeno S. 2009. The Inhibitory effect on aldose reductase by an extract of Ganoderma lucidum. Phytother Res 23: 28–32.

Fatmawati S, Shimizu K, Kondo R. 2010a. Ganoderic acid Df, a new triterpenoid with aldose reductase inhibitory activity from the fruiting body of Ganoderma lucidum Fitoterapia 81: 1033-1036.

Fatmawati S, Shimizu K, Kondo R. 2010b. Inhibition of aldose reductase in vitro by constituents of Ganoderma lucidum. Planta Med 76: 1691-1693.

Fuente DL, Manzanaro S, Martín MJ et al. 2003. Synthesis, activity, and molecular modeling studies of novel human aldose reductase inhibitors based on a marine natural product. J Med Chem 46: 5208–5221.

Fujita T, Ohira K, Miyatake K et al. 1995. Inhibitory effect of perilloside A and C, and related monoterpene glucoside on aldose reductase and their structure activity relationship. Chem Pharm Bull 43: 920-926.

Gacche RN, Dhole NA. 2011a. Aldose reductase inhibitory, anti-cataract and antioxidant potential of selected medicinal plants from the Marathwada region, India. Nat Prod Res 25: 760–763.

Gacche RN, Dhole NA. 2011b. Profie of aldose reductase inhibition, anti-cataract and free radical scavenging activity of selected medicinal plants: An attempt to standardize the botanicals for amelioration of diabetes complications. Fod Chem Toxicol 49: 1806-1813.

Goodarzi MT, Zal F, Malakooti M et al.. 2006. Inhibitory activity of flavonoids on the lens aldose reductase of healthy and diabetic rats. Acta Medica Iranica 44: 41-45.

Guzmán A, Ricardo OG. 2005. Inhibition of aldose reductase by herbs extract and natural substance and their role in prevention of cataracts. Rev Cubana Plant Med 10: 3-4.

Halder N, Joshi S, Gupta SK. 2003. Lens aldose reductase inhibiting potential of some indigenous plants. J Ethanopharmacol 86: 113-116.

Haraguchi H, Hayashi R, Ishizu T et al. 2003. A flavone from Manilkara indica as a specific inhibitor against aldose reductase in vitro. Planta Med 69: 853-855.

Haraguchi H, Ohmi I, Fukuda A et al. 1997. Inhibition of aldose reductase and sorbitol accumulation by astilbin and toxifolin dihydroflavonols in Engelhardtia chrysolepis. Biosci Biotechnol Biochem 61: 651-54.

Haraguchi H, Ohmi I, Sakai S et al. 1996. Effect of Polygonum hydropiper sulfated flavonoids on lens aldose reductase and related enzyme. J Nat Prod 59: 443-445.

Hayman S, Kinoshita JH. 1965. Isolation and properties of lens Aldose reductase. J Biol Chem.240: 877-882.

Hong Mei Li, Seung Hwan Hwang, Beom Goo Kang, Jae Seung Hong, Soon Sung Lim. Inhibitory Effects of Colocasia esculenta (L.) Schott Constituents on Aldose Reductase. Molecules. 2014; 19: 13212-13224.

Hsieh P-C, Huang G-J, Ho Y-L et al. 2010. Activities of antioxidants, α-Glucosidase inhibitors and aldose reductase inhibitors of the aqueous extracts of four Flemingia species in Taiwan. Bot Studies 51: 293-302.

International Diabetes Federation (IDF), Diabetes Atlas Seventh Edition 2015.

Jung HA, Islam MD, Kwon YS et al. 2011. Extraction and identification of three major aldose reductase inhibitors from Artemisia Montana. Food Chem Toxicol 49: 376–384.

Jung HA, Jung YJ, Yoon NY et al. 2008a. Inhibitory effect of Nelumbo nucifera leaves on rat lens aldose reductase, advanced glycation endproducts formation and oxidative stress. Food Chem Toxicol 46: 3818-3826.

Jung HA, Kim YS, Choi JS. 2009. Quantitative HPLC analysis of two key flavonoids and inhibitory activities against aldose reductase from different parts of the Korean thistle, Cirsiummaackii. Food Cheml Toxicol 47: 2790–2797.

Jung HA, Yoon NY, Kang SS et al. 2008b. Inhibitory activities of prenylated flavonoids from Sophora flavescens against aldose reductase and generation of advanced glycation endproducts. J Pharm Pharmacol 60: 1227-1236.

Jung SH, Lee JM, Lee HJ et al. 2007. Aldose reductase and advanced glycation endproducts inhibitory effect of Phyllostachys nigra. Biol Pharma Bull 30(8): 1569-1572.

Jung SH, Lee YS, Lee S et al. 2002. Isoflavonoids from the rhizomes of Belamcanda chinensis and their effect on aldose reductase and sorbitol accumulation in streptozotocin induced diabetic rat tissues. Arch Pharma Res 3: 306-312.

Kador PF, Kinoshita JH, Tung WH et al. 1980. Differences in the susceptibility of various aldose reductases to inhibition. Invest Opthalmol Visual Sci 19: 980-982.

Kaoru A , Masato T, Hideo S, Toshiinasa O, Hiroshi S,Hiroaki N, Masao C, and Hiroshi M. 1989 The Existence of Aldose Reductase Inhibitors in Some Kampo Medicines (Oriental Herb Prescriptions). Planta Medica 55, 409-38.

Kasimu R, Basnet P, Tezuka Y et al.1997. Danshenols A and B, new aldose reductase inhibitors from the roots of Salvia miltiorhiza. Chem Pharm Bull 45: 564-566.

Kato A, Higuchi Y, Gato H et al. 2006. Inhibitory effects of Zingiber officinale Roscoe derived components on aldose reductase activity in vitro and in vivo. J Agric Food Chem 54: 6640-6644.

Kato A, Yasuko H, Goto H et al. 2009. Inhibitory effect of rhetsinine isolated from Evodia rutaecarpa on aldose reductase activity. Phytomedicine 16: 258-261.

Kawanishi K, Ueda H, Moriyasu M. 2003. Aldose reductase inhibitors from nature. Curr Med Chem 10: 1353-1374.

Kim J, Kim CS, Sohn E et al. 2011. KIOM-79 inhibits aldose reductase activity and cataractogenesis in Zucker diabetic fatty rats. J Pharm Pharmacol 63: 1301–1308.

Kim JH, Ryu YB, Kang NS et al. 2006. Glycosidase inhibitory flavonoids from Sophora flavescens. Biol Phrama Bull 29: 302-305.

Kodha H, Tanaka S, Yamaoka Y et al.1989. Studies on lens- aldose- reductase inhibitor in medicinal plants. II. active constituents of Monochsma savatierii. Chem Pharm Bull 37: 3153-3154.

Koukoulitsa C, Zika C, Geromichalos GD et al. 2006. Evaluation of aldose reductase inhibition and docking studies of some secondary metabolites, isolated from Origanum vulgare L. ssp. Hirtum. Bioorg Med Chem 14: 1653-1659.

Kubo M, Matsuda H, Tokuoka K et al. 1994. Studies of anti-cataract drugs from natural sources.I. Effects of methanolic extract and the alkaloidal components from Corydalis Tuber on in vitro aldose reductase activity. Biol Pharm Bull 17: 458-459.

Lee EH, Song DG, Lee JY et al. 2008. Inhibitory effect of the compounds isolated from Rhus verniciflua on aldose reductase and advanced glycation endproducts. Biol Pharma Bull 31(8): 1626-1630.

Lee HS. 2002a. Inhibitory activity of Cinnamomum cassia bark derived component against rat lens aldose reductase. J Pharm Pharmaceut Sci 5: 226-230.

Lee HS. 2005. Cuminaldehyde: Aldose reductase and α-glucosidase inhibitor derived from Cuminum cyminum L.seeds. J Agric Food Chem 53: 2446-2450.

Lee HS.2002b. Rat lens aldose reductase inhibitory activities of Coptis japonica root derived isoquiniline alkaloids. J Agric Food Chem 50: 7013-7016.

Lee S, Jung SH, Lee YS et al. 2002. Coumarins from Angelica gigas roots having rat lens aldose reductase activity. J Appl Pharmacol 10: 85-88.

Lee S, Shim SH, Kim JS et al. 2005. Aldose reductase inhibitors from the fruiting bodies of Ganoderma applanatum. Biol Pharma Bull 28(6): 1103-1105.

Lee SJ, Park WH, Park SD et al. 2009. Aldose reductase inhibitors from Litchi chinensis Sonn. J Enzyme Inhib Med Chem 24(4): 957-959.

Lee YS, Kim JK, Bae YS et al. 2011. Inhibitory effect of glucodistylin from the bark of Quercus acutissima on human recombinant aldose reductase and sorbitol accumulation. Arch Pharm Res 34: 211-215.

Lee YS, Kim SH, Jung SH et al. 2010. Aldose reductase inhibitory compounds from Glycyrrhiza uralensis. Biol Phrama Bull 33(5): 917-921.

Lim SS, Jung YJ, Hyum SK et al. 2006. Rat lens aldose reductase inhibitory constituents of Nelumbo nucifera stamens. Phytother Res 20: 825-830.

Logendra S, Ribnicky DM, Yang H et al. 2006. Bioassay guided isolation of aldose reductase inhibitors from Artemisia dracunculus. Phytochemistry 67: 1539-1546.

Manzanaro S, Salva J, Angel de la Fuente J et al. 2006. Phenolic marine natural products as aldose reductase inhibitors. J Nat Prod 69: 1485-1487.

Matsuda H, Morikawa T, Toguchida I et al. 2002a. Medicinal flowers. Part VI. Absolute stereostructures of two new flavonone glycosides(I) and a phenylbutanoid glycoside(II) from the flowers of Chrysanthem indicum: Their inhibitory activities for rat lens aldose reductase. Chem Pharm Bull 50: 972-975.

Matsuda H, Morikawa T, Toguchida I et al. 2002b.Structural requirements of flavonoids and related compounds for aldose reductase inhibitory activity. Chem Pharm Bull 50:788-795.

Matsuda H, Murakami T, Yashiro K et al.1999. Antidiabetic principles of natural medicines. IV. Aldose Reductase and α-glucosidase inhibitors from the roots of Salacia oblonga Wall. (Celastraceae): Structure of a new friedelane-type triterpene, kotalagenin 16-acetate. Chem Pharm Bull 47: 1725-1729.

Moghaddam MS, Kumar PA, Reddy GB et al. 2005. Effect of diabecon on sugar induced lens opacity in organ culture: mechanism of action. J Ethnopharmacol 97: 397-403.

Moon HI, Jung JC, Lee J. 2006. Aldose reductase inhibitory effect by tectorigenin derivatives from Viola hondoensis. Biorg Med Chem 14: 7592-7594.

Morikawa T, Kishi A, Pongpiriyadacha Y et al. 2003. Structures of new friedelane type triterpenes and eudesmane type sesqiterpene and aldose reductase inhibitors from Salacia chinensis. J Nat Prod 66: 1191-1196.

Morikawa T, Xie H, Wang T et al. 2008. Bioactive constituents from Chinese Natural Medicines xxxvii. Aminopeptidase N and Aldose reductase Inhibitors from Sinocrassula indica: structures of sinocrassosides B4, B5, C1, and D1-D3. Chem Pharm Bull 56: 1438-1444.

Murata M, Iries J, Homma S et al. 1994. Aldose reductase inhibitors from green tea. Lebensm Wiss u Technol 27: 401-405.

Muthenna P, Suryanarayana P, Gunda SK et al. 2009. Inhibition of aldose reductase by dietary antioxidant curcumin: Mechanism of inhibition, specificity and significance. FEBS Lett 583: 3637–3642.

Nishimura.C, Yamaoka T, Mizutani M et al. 1991. Purification and characterization of the recombinant human Aldose reductase expressed in baculovirus system.Biochem Biophys Acta 1078: 171-178.

Ohkubo Y, Kishikawa H, Araki E et al. 1995. Intensive insulin therapy prevents the progression of diabetic microvascular complications in Japanese patients with non-insulin-dependent diabetes mellitus: arandomized prospective 6-year study. Diabetes Res Clin Pract 28: 103-117.

Okada Y, Miyauchi N, Suzuki K et al. 1995. Search for naturally occurring substances to prevent the complication of diabetes.II.Inhibitory effect of coumarin and flavonoid derivatives on bovine lens aldose reductase and rabbit platelet aggregation. Chem Pharm Bull 43: 1385-1387.

Park C-H, Lim SS, Lee D-U. 2007. Structure activity relationships of components from the roots of Pueraria thunbergiana having aldose reductase inhibitory and antioxidative activity. Bull Korean Chem Soc 28: 493-495.

Park HY, Kwon SB, Heo NK et al. 2011. Constituents of the stem of Angelica gigas with rat lens aldose reductase inhibitory activity. J Korean Soc Appl Biol Chem 54: 194-199.

Patel DK, Kumar R, Kumar M et al. 2012. Evaluation of in vitro aldose reductase inhibitory potential of different fraction of Hybanthus enneaspermus Linn F. Muell. Asian Pac J Trop Biomed 2: 134-139.

Peyroux J, Sternberg M. 2006. Advanced glycation end products (AGEs): pharmacological inhibition in diabetes. Pathol Biol 54: 405-419.

Rosler KH, Goodwin RS, Mabry TJ et al.1984. Flavonoids with anti cataract activity from Brickellia arguta. J Nat Prod 47: 316-319.

Sakai I, Izumi SI, Murano T et al. 2001. Presence of aldose reductase inhibitors in tea leaves. Jpn J Pharmacol 85: 322-326.

Saraswat M, Muthenna P, Suryanarayana P et al. 2008. Dietary sources of aldose reductase inhibitors: prospects for alleviating diabetic complications. Asia Pac J Clin Nutr 17: 558-565.

Sato S, Takeo J, Aoyama C et al. 2007. Na+-glucose cotransporter (SGLT) inhibitory flavonoids from the roots of Sophora flavescens. Bioorg med chem 15: 3445-3449.

Suryanarayana P, Saraswat M, Mrudula T et al. 2005. Curcumin and turmeric delay streptozotocin-induced diabetic cataract in rats. Invest Ophthalmol Vis Sci 46: 2092–2099.

Surynarayana P, Kumar PA, Sarasawat M et al. 2004. Inhibition of aldose reductase by tannoid principles of Emblica officinalis: Implications for the prevention of sugar cataract. Mol Vis 10: 148-154.

Terashima S, Shimizu M, Nakayama H, Ishikura M, Ueda Y, Imai K, Suzui A, Morita N.1990.Studies on aldose reductase inhibitors from medicinal plant of "sinfito," Potentilla candicans, and further synthesis of their related compounds. Chem. Pharm bull; 38(10):2733-6.

Termentzi A, Alexiou P, Demopoulos VJ et al. 2008. The aldose reductase inhibitory capacity of Sorbus domestica fruit extracts depends on their phenolic content and may be useful for the control of diabetic complications. Pharmazie 63: 693-696.

Tomás-Barberán FA, Lopez GC, Villar A et al.1986. Inhibition of lens aldose reductase by Labiatae flavonoids. Planta Med 6: 239-240.

Toyomizu M, Sugiyama S, Jin RL, Nakatsu T. 1993. α-Glucosidase and Aldose Reductase Inhibitors: Constituents of Cashew, Anacardium occidentale, Nut Shell Liquids. Phytotherapy research, 7, 252-254.

Ueda H, Kuroiwa E, Tachibana Y et al. 2004. Aldose reductase inhibitors from the leaves of Myrciaria dubia. Phytomedicine 11: 652-656.

Varma SD, Kinoshita JH. 1976. Inhibition of lens aldose reductase by flavonoides –their possible role in the prevention of diabetic cataracts. Biochem Pharma 25: 2505-2513.

Varma SD, Mikuni I, Kinoshita JH et al.1975. Flavonoids as inhibitors of lens aldose reductase. Science 188: 1215-1216.

Wirasathien L, Pengsuparp T, Suttisri R et al. 2007. Inhibitors of aldose reductase and advanced glycation end products formation from the leaves of Stelechocarpus cauliflorus. Phytomedicine 14: 546-550.

Xie H, Wang T, Matsuda H et al. 2005. Bioactive constituents from Chinese natural medicine.XV.Inhibitory effect on aldose reductase and structure of saussureosides A and B from Saussurea medusa. Chem Pharm Bull 53: 1416-1422.

Xu Z, Yang H, Zhou M et al. 2010. Inhibitory effect of total lignan from Fructus Arctii on aldose reductase. Phytother Res 24: 472–473.

Yawadio R, Shinji T, Naofumi M. 2006. Identification of phenolic compounds isolated from pigmented rices and their aldose reductase inhibitory activities. Food Chem 101: 1616-1625.

Yoshikawa M, Morikawa T, Murakami T et al. 1999. Medicinal flowers.I.Aldose reductase inhibitors and three new eudesmane type sesquiterpenes, kikkanols A, B, and C, from the flower of Chrysanthem indicum. Chem Pharm Bull 47: 340-345.

Yoshikawa M, Murakami T, Ishiwada T et al. 2002. New flavonol oligoglycosides and polyacylated sucroses with inhibitory effects on aldose reductase and platelet aggregation from the flowers of Prunus mume. J Nat Prod 65: 1151-1155.

Yoshikawa M, Shimada H, Nishida N et al. 1998. Antidiabetic principles of natural medicines.II. Aldose reductase and α-glucosidase inhibitors from Brazilian natural medicine, the leaves of Myrcia multiflora DC. (Myrtaceae):structures of myrciaphenones A and B. Chem Pharm Bull 46: 113-119.

Zhiqiang Wang, Seung Hwan Hwang, Yanymee N. Guillen Quispe, Paul H. Gonzales Arce, Soon Sung Lim. Investigation of the antioxidant and aldose reductase inhibitory activities of extracts from Peruvian tea plant infusions. Food Chemistry 231 (2017) 222–230.

Chapter 2

Aldose Reductase Inhibitors from Plant Extracts

In previous chapter, we discussed the importance of aldose reductase enzyme in diabetic complications. And also describe about phytochemicals how they inhibit the AR. Here we also give the details about different plant extracts how the influence on inhibitory activity of AR using deferent assay methods.

Four Indian plants viz. *Ocimum sanctum* (OS; Tulsi), *Curcuma longa* (CL; Haldi), *Withania somnifera* (WS; Ashwagandha) and *Azadirachta indica* (AI; Neem) were selected to evaluate their AR inhibiting capacity. All the four plants were found to inhibit lens AR activity but to different extent. From dose–response curve, OS was found to be the most effective AR inhibitor followed by CL, AI and WS. The plants relied on their reported hypoglycemic activity. Also, they are commonly consumed in the diet or used as home remedies in various pathological conditions (Halder *et al.*, 2003).

The water, ethanol and chloroform extracts of selected plants such as *Adhatoda vasica* (L.) (Acanthaceae), *Caesalpinia bonduc* (L.), *Cassia fistula* (L.) (Caesalpiniaceae) and *Biophytum sensitivum* (L.) (Oxalidaceae) were evaluated for rat lens aldose reductase inhibitory (RLAR) potential. All the samples inhibited the aldose reductase considerably. C. fistula (IC50, 0.154 mgmL1) showed significant RLAR inhibitory activity as compared to the other tested samples. (Gacche *et al.*, 2011a).

In another study, different fractions of *Catharanthus roseus L.* (Apocynaceae), *Ocimum sanctum L.* (Labiatae), *Tinospora cordifolia Willd.* (Menispermaceae), *Aegle marmelos L.* (Rutaceae), *Ficus glomerata L.* (Moraceae), *Psoralea corlifolia L.* (Fabaceae), *Tribulus terrestris L.* (Zygophyllaceae), and *Morinda cetrifolia L.* (Rubiaceae) were evaluated as possible inhibitors of aldose reductase. Among the tested plants, water extract of *M.citrifolia* (IC50 0.132 mg/mL) exhibited maximum AR inhibitory activity as compared toother phyto fractions which showed the activity in an IC50 range of 0.176–0.0.82 mg/mL. (Gacche *et al.*, 2011b).

Different fractions of *Hybanthus enneaspermus* were found to inhibit rat lens aldose reductase activity to various extents with IC_{50} values ranging from 2 µg/mL to >100 µg/mL. The aldose reductase activity in normal rat lens was found to be (0.0144±0.0007 µg/mL). Among the fractions, ethyl acetate fraction showed higher percentage of inhibition (IC_{50} (49.26±1.76 µg/mL) followed by aqueous fraction (IC_{50} 70.83±2.82 µg/mL). Chloroform fraction (IC50 (98.52±1.80 µg/mL) also showed significant inhibition but was less as compared with the ethyl acetate fraction. Petroleum ether fraction (IC_{50} 118.89±0.71 µg/mL) was found to have the least inhibition potential against aldose reductase enzyme (Patel *et al.*, 2012).

The aqueous extracts of 22 plant-derived materials were prepared and evaluated for the inhibitory property against rat lens and human recombinant aldose reductase. Specificity of these extracts towards aldose reductase was established by testing their ability to inhibit a closely related enzyme *viz*, aldehyde reductase. Among the 22 dietary sources tested, 10 showed considerable inhibitory potential against both rat lens and human recombinant aldose reductase. Prominent inhibitory property was found in spinach, cumin, fennel, lemon, basil and black pepper with an approximate IC_{50} of 0.2 mg/mL with an excellent selectivity towards aldose reductase. As against this, 10 to 20 times higher concentrations were required for 50% inhibition of aldehyde reductase (Saraswat *et al.*, 2008).

The human aldose reductase inhibitory effects of the methanol extracts of 17 medicinal and edible mushrooms were examined. *Ganoderma lucidum* showed the highest aldose reductase inhibitory activity compared with the other mushrooms. The effect of an ethanol extract of *G. lucidum* on the galactitol level in the eye lens was studied in a galactosemic rat model *in vivo*. This mushroom significantly decreased the galactitol accumulation (Fatmawati *et al.*, 2009).

KIOM-79, a combination of four plant extracts, has a preventive effect on diabetic nephropathy and retinopathy in diabetic animal models. KIOM-79 was tested for its effect on an *in-vitro* aldose reductase activity assay. The IC_{50} values of KIOM-79 in this assay were compared with a known aldose reductase inhibitor 3,3-tetramethyleneglutaric acid (Table 2.1). KIOM-79 had an apparent inhibitory effect on aldose reductase activity (IC_{50} value 10.09 mg/mL) (Kim *et al.*, 2011).

Table 2.1 Plant extracts with aldose reductase (AR) inhibitory activities.

S.No.	Extract	Family	Part used	Solvent used	IC$_{50}$ (µg/mL)		Reference
					RLAR	**HRAR**	
1.	*Azadirachta indica*	Meliaceae	LF	H$_2$O	57		Halder *et al.*, 2003
	Curcuma longa	Zingiberaceae	RZ	"	55		"
	Ocimum sanctum	Lamiaceae	LF	"	20		"
	Withania somnifera	Solanaceae	RT	"	89		"
2.	*Embelica officinalis*	Phyllanthaceae	FT	H$_2$O	720	880	Surynarayana *et al.*, 2004
	E. officinalis tannoids		"		6.1	9.8	
3.	[R]Diabecon			H$_2$O	10	-	Moghaddam *et al.*, 2005
	Gymnema sylvestre	Ascelpidaceae	WP	"	16	-	
4.	*Aralia elata*	Araliaceae	CX	H$_2$O	11.3	-	Chung *et al.*, 2005
5.	*Curcuma longa*	Zingiberaceae	RZ	EtOH	75%*		Guzmán *et al.*, 2005
	Eugenia borinquensis	Myrtaceae		EtOH	82%		"
	Eucalyptus deglupta	Myrtaceae		EtOH	88%		"
	Mangifera indica	Anacardiaceae		EtOH	92%		"
	Syzygium malaccense			EtOH	82%		"
	Vaccinium myttillus	Ericaceae		EtOH	67%		"
6.	*Arctium lappa* L. total lignan (200 µg/mL)	Asteraceae	RFT	-	90%		Xu *et al.*, 2010
7.	*Hybanthus enneaspermus*	Violaceae	NI	H$_2$O	70.83± 2.82		Patel *et al.*, 2012
			NI	EtOAc	49.26± 1.76		"
			NI	CHCl$_3$	98.52±1.80		"
			NI	Pet eher	118.89±0.71		"

Table 2.1 Contd...

S.No.	Extract	Family	Part used	Solvent used	IC$_{50}$ (µg/mL)		Reference
					RLAR	HRAR	
8.	*KIOM-79			80% methanol	10.09±0.573		Kim *et al.*, 2011
9.	*Agaricus bisporus*	Agaricaceae	FTB	MeOH	~17%		Fatmawati *et al.*, 2009
	Agaricus blazei Murr	Agaricaceae	"	"	~27%		"
	Agrocybe cylindracea (DC.:Fr.) Maire.	Bolbitiaceae	"	"	~6%		"
	Flammulina velutipes (Curt.:Fr.) Sing.	Tricholomataceae	"	"	~14%		"
	Ganoderma lucidum	Ganodermataceae	"	"	~84%		"
	Grifora fondosa (Dicks.:Fr.) S. F. Gray	Polyporaceae	"	"	~36%		"
	Hericium erinaceum (Fr.) Pers.	Hericiaceae	"	"	~13%		"
	Hypoloma sublateritium (Fr.) Quel	Strophariaceae	"	"	~58%		"
	Hypsizygus marmoreus (Peck) Bigelow	Tricholomataceae	"	"	~27%		"
	Lentinula edodes (Berk.) Pegler ()	Trichloromataceae	"	"	~30%		"
	Lyophyllum decastes (Fr.:Fr.) Sing ()	Tricholoromataceae	"	"	~12%		"
	Panellus serotinus (Pers.:Fr.) Kuhn. (),	Tricholomataceae	"	"	~30%		"

Table 2.1 *Contd...*

S.No.	Extract	Family	Part used	Solvent used	IC$_{50}$ (µg/mL)		Reference
					RLAR	HRAR	
	Pleurotus abalonus Han, K. M. Chen et S. Cheng	Pleurotaceae	"	"	~12%		"
	Pleurotus comucopiae (Paulet) Rolland var. *citrinopileatus* (Sing) Ohira	Pleurotaceae	"	"	~54%		"
	Pleurotus eringii (De Candolle:Fr.) Quel.	(Pleurotaceae)	"	"	~32%		"
	Pleurotus ostreatus (Jacq.:Fr.) Kummer	Pleurotaceae	"	"	~34%		"
	Pholiota nameko (T. Ito) S. Ito et Imai in Imai	Strophariaceae	"	"	~20%		"
10.	*Spinaceae oleracea* (Spinach)		LF	H$_2$O	0.10 ± 0.01	0.11 ± 0.005	Saraswat *et al.* 2008
	Cuminum cyminum (Cumin)		SD	"	0.17 ± 0.02	0.15 ± 0.01	"
	Foeniculum vulgare (Fennel)	Apiaceae	SD	"	0.18 ± 0.02	0.19 ± 0.02	"
	Ocimum sanctum (Basil)	Lamiaceae	LF	"	0.20 ± 0.01	0.12 ± 0.01	"
	Piper nigrum (Black pepper)	Piperaceae	SD	"	0.22 ± 0.02	0.22 ± 0.03	"
	Trigonella foenumgraceum (Fenugreek)	Trigonalaceae	SD	"	0.24 ± 0.03	0.30 ± 0.03	"
	Citrus lemon Lemon	Rutaceae	FT	"	0.25 ± 0.01	0.18 ± 0.01	"
	Momordica charantia (Bitter gourd)	Cucurbitaceae	FT	"	0.28 ± 0.02	0.25 ± 0.01	"

Table 2.1 *Contd...*

S.No.	Extract	Family	Part used	Solvent used	IC$_{50}$ (µg/mL)		Reference
					RLAR	HRAR	
	Citrus aurantium var. sinensis (Orange)	Rutaceae	FT	”	0.28 ± 0.04	0.25 ± 0.02	”
	Murraya koenigii Curry leaves		LF	”	0.31± 0.01	0.28 ± 0.03	”
	Cinamomum zeylencium (Cinnamon)		BK	”	0.4 ± 0.02	0.19 ± 0.02	”
	Trachyspermum ammi (Ajwain)		SD	”	0.65 ± 0.03	N.T.	”
	Psidium guajava (Gauva Fruit)		FT	”	0.70 ± 0.03	N.T.	”
	Flemingia lineata (L.) Roxb. (FL)				269.66 ± 0.40		Hsieh *et al.*, 2010
	F. macrophylla (Willd.) Kuntze *ex* Prain (FM)				153.92 ± 0.20		
	F. prostrata Roxb (FP)				1091.91 ± 1.63		
	F. strobilifera (L.) R. Br. Ex Ait. (FS)				1468.60 ± 2.10		
	Artemisia apiacea (Hance)	Asteraceae	WP	MeOH	0.67 ± 0.05	N.T.	Jung *et al.*, 2011
	A. argyi Levi. et Vaniot		LF	”	4.83 ± 0.90	N.T.	”
	A. capillaris Thunb.		WP	”	3.94 ± 0.18	N.T.	”
	A. iwayomogi Kitamura WP		WP	”	0.74 ± 0.09	N.T.	”
	A. japonica Thunb. WP		WP	”	1.13 ± 0.24	N.T.	”
	A. keiskeana Miq. WP		WP	”	5.64 ± 0.00	N.T.	”

Table 2.1 *Contd…*

S.No.	Extract	Family	Part used	Solvent used	IC$_{50}$ (µg/mL)		Reference
					RLAR	HRAR	
	A. montana Pampan		WP	”	0.51 ± 0.06	N.T.	”
	A. princeps var. orientalis Pampan		WP	”	13.45 ± 2.57	N.T.	”
	A. rubripes Nakai		WP	”	0.61 ± 0.13	N.T.	”
	A. selengensis Turcz		WP	”	3.67 ± 0.16	N.T.	”
	A. stolonifera Max.		WP	”	4.60 ± 0.32	N.T.	”
	A. sylvatica Max.		WP	”	1.01 ± 0.18	N.T.	”
	A. vasica (L.)	Acanthaceae		H$_2$O			Gacche and Dhole, 2011a
				EtOH			”
				CHCl$_3$			”
	Cassia fistula (L.)	Caesalpiniaceae		H$_2$O			”
				EtOH			”
				CHCl$_3$	154		”
	Caesalpinia bonduc (L.)	Caesalpiniaceae		H$_2$O			”
				EtOH			”
				CHCl$_3$			”
	Biophytum sensitivum	Oxalidaceae		H$_2$O			”
				EtOH			”
				CHCl$_3$			”
	Aegle marmelos L	Rutaceae		H$_2$O	403		Gacche and Dhole, 2011b
				EtOH	766		
				CHCl$_3$	810		
	Catharnthus roseus L.	Apocyanaceae		H$_2$O	342		
				EtOH	300		

Table **2.1** Contd...

S.No.	Extract	Family	Part used	Solvent used	IC$_{50}$ (µg/mL)		Reference
					RLAR	HRAR	
				CHCl$_3$	820		
	Ficus golmerata L.	Moraceae		H$_2$O	310		
				EtOH	300		
				CHCl$_3$	762		
	Morinda certifolia L.	Rubiaceae		H$_2$O	132		
				EtOH	242		
				CHCl$_3$	520		
	Ocimum sanctum L.	Lamiaceae		H$_2$O	280		
				EtOH	320		
				CHCl$_3$	350		
	Psoralea corlifolia L.	Fabaceae		H$_2$O	286		
				EtOH	292		
				CHCl$_3$	318		
	Tinospora cordifolia Willd	Menispermaceae		H$_2$O	210		
				EtOH	176		
				CHCl$_3$	328		
	Tribulus terrestris L.	Zygophyllaceae		H$_2$O	348		
				EtOH	368		
				CHCl$_3$	444		

[*] KIOM is the 80% ethanol extract mixture of the radix of *Euphorbia pekinensis,* radix of *Glycyrrhiza uralensis,* gingered *Magnolia officinalis* cortex, and parched radix of *Pueraria lobata.*

In order to evaluate the AR inhibitory activity, the MeOH extracts of different species were tested via the RLAR inhibition assay. The RLAR inhibitory activities of the selected twelve species of the genus Artemisia are summarized in the Table 2.1. All species showed predominant and concentration-dependent inhibitory activities, but to a different extent with IC_{50} values ranging from 0.51 to 13.45 µg/mL. Among them, the MeOH extract of the whole plant of *A. montana* showed the highest inhibitory activity with an IC_{50} value of 0.51 ± 0.06 µg/mL, compared to the positive control, quercetin, with an IC_{50} value of 0.64 ± 0.09 µg/mL. *A. rubripes*, *A. apiacea*, and *A. iwayomogi* also showed significant inhibitory activities with IC_{50} values of 0.61 ± 0.13, 0.67 ± 0.05, and 0.74 ± 0.09 µg/mL, respectively. The RLAR inhibitory activities were also displayed by *A. sylvatica* and *A. japonica*, with the respective IC_{50} values of 1.01 ± 0.18 and 1.13 ± 0.24 µg/mL, followed by *A. selengenis*, *A. capillaris*, *A. stolonifera*, *A. argyi*, and *A. keiskeana* with IC_{50} values ranging from 3.67 to 5.64 µg/mL, while *A. princeps* var. orientalis exhibited a moderate RLAR inhibitory activity with an IC_{50} value of 13.45 ± 2.57 µg/mL (Jung *et al.*, 2011).

Diabecon is inhibited AR with an IC50 value of 10µg/mL (±1.8; $n = 3$) where as its ethanol, ethyl acetate extracts did not show considerable inhibition. Since Diabecon is a polyherbal combination, one or all of the constituent herbs may be responsible for AR inhibition. They assessed AR inhibitory potential of three potential herbs, *Gymnema sylvestre*, *Eugenia jambolana* and *Gmelina arborea*, out of a dozen herbs used for Diabecon preparation. Aqueous extract of *Gymnema sylvestre* showed significant AR inhibition with an IC_{50} value of 16µg/mL (±2.1; $n=3$), other two plants fail to show significant inhibition (Moghaddama *et al.*, 2005).

The potent inhibitory effect of the total lignan from the plant *Fructus arctii* on aldose reductase was observed, the *Fructus* exhibited nearly the same AR inhibitory activity as that of Epalrestat at concentrations of 200 µg/mL. It was obvious that *Fructus* possesses inhibitory activity on AR at the reported concentrations and in a dose-dependent manner (Xu *et al.*, 2010).

The water extract of *Aralia elata* (*Aralia* extract) has been used in Korean traditional medicine to treat diabetes mellitus. Here, we investigated. The inhibitory activity of *Aralia* extract on AR activity was determined in an *in vitro* system. The resulting IC_{50} value of *Aralia* extract was found to be11.3µg/mL (Chung *et al.*, 2005).

As it is shown in the Figure 2.1, the diethyl ether and ethyl acetate fractions isolated from *Sorbus domestica* fruits exhibited high ALR2 inhibitory activity at a final concentration of 50 mg/mL ranging from 72 to 93%. Among the diethyl ether extracts of the five different categories of the fruits, the raw yellow fruits were the strongest inhibitors (93% at 50 mg/mL). Interestingly, this fruit category has shown no significant difference in ALR2 inhibitory activity from those fruits left to mature for either 1 or 3 weeks as well as those that are well matured on the trees (86%, 85% and 86%, respectively, at 50 mg/mL). On the contrary, the fruit pulp exhibited the lowest, but still significant inhibitory activity (72% at 50 mg/mL). Regarding the ethyl acetate fraction, the different maturity stages of the fruits do not seem to affect their ALR2 inhibitory activity (ranging 80–86% at 50 mg/mL). Furthermore, the dichloromethane fractions possessed inhibitory activity above 50%. In comparison, those of the well-matured fruits on the trees and those collected unripe and left to mature for either 1 or 3 weeks at room temperature, the ALR2 inhibitory activity appears weak below 40% for the butanol and water extracts as well as for the residues (Termentzi *et al.*, 2008).

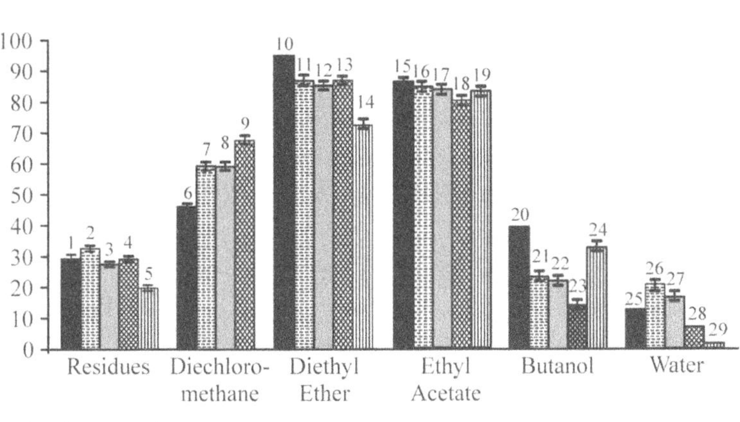

Figure 2.1 Inhibitory effect of Sorbus domestica fruits' extracts on aldose reductase Enzyme (in final concentration that of 50 ml). (Termentzi *et al.,* 2008).

E. officinalis extract inhibited rat lens and recombinant human AR with IC50 values 0.72 and 0.88 mg/mL respectively. Since *E. officinalis* is a rich source of ascorbic acid, so and investigated whether ascorbic acid was responsible for AR inhibition by *E. officinalis* extract. However, ascorbic acid did not inhibit AR even at 5 mM concentration. Further, we demonstrate that the hydrolysable tannoids of *E. officinalis* were responsible for AR inhibition, as enriched tannoids of *E. officinalis* exhibited remarkable inhibition against both rat lens and human AR with IC_{50} of 6 and 10 microg/mL respectively. The inhibition of AR by *E. officinalis* tannoids is 100 times higher than its aqueous extract and comparable to or better than quercetin (Surynarayana *et al.*, 2004).

13 plants and 3 natural products were randomly selected for experiment. The 19 extracts originated from plant material which was extracted with ethanol, water and DCM, and assessed for inhibitors of aldose reductase. Among the three evaluated natural products, C. longa, known as turmeric (75%), and the EtOH extract of *V. myrtillus* known as bilberry (67%), were found to have the best inhibitory activity. The plant extracts of *Eugenia borinquensis* (82%), *Eucalyptus deglupta* (88%), and *Mangifera indica* (92%) were among the best inhibitors of aldose reductase (Guzmán *et al.*, 2005).

Aqueous extracts of *Flemingia macrophylla (Willd.)* Kuntze exPrain (FM), *Flemingia prostrate Roxb (FP)*, *Flemingia lineate (L.)* Roxb. (FL), and *Flemingia strobilifera (L.)* R. Br. Ex Ait. (FS) evaluated the inhibitory activity on AR. Flemingia species AR inhibitory activities ranged from 79.36 μg/mL to 172.41 μg/mL, and increased as in the following order: WFM > WFS > WFL> WFP. WFM had the highest AR inhibitory activity (IC_{50}= 79.36 ± 3.20 μg/mL). The positive control in the AR inhibitory activity assay was genistein (IC_{50}= 45.62 ± 2.16 μg/mL) (Hsieh *et al.*, 2010).

Pomegranate ethanolic seed and hull extracts were tested, in comparison with a commercial sample, for the inhibition of aldose reductase. Pomegranate ethanolic hull extract and commercial pomegranate hull extract exhibited similar aldose reductase inhibitory activity characterized by IC50 values ranging from 3 to 33.3 μg/mL. They were more effective than pomegranate ethanolic seed extract with IC50 ranging from 33.3 to 333 μg/mL (Karasu *et al.*, 2012).

Gentiana lutea grows naturally in the central and southern areas of Europe. Its roots are commonly consumed as a beverage in some European countries and are also known to have medicinal properties. The water, ethanol, methanol, and ether extracts of the roots of *G. lutea* were subjected to *in vitro* bioassay to evaluate their inhibitory activity on the ALR2. While the ether and methanol extracts showed greater inhibitory activities against both rat lens and human ALR2, the water and ethanol extracts showed moderate inhibitory activities (Akileshwari *et al.*, 2012).

The alcoholic extract of *Ceasalpinia digyna* and *Alangium lamarckii* had a potent inhibitory effect on the lens AR enzyme. The IC_{50} values of alcoholic extract of the selected plants were calculated and were (46.29±11.17) and (106.00±5.11) μg/mL, respectively. Quercetin was used as a positive control and its IC$_{50}$ value was (2.95±1.53) µg/ml (Rajesh *et al.,* 2011).

Four standardized plant extracts used for the treatment of diabetes and related diseases, and their principal components for AR inhibitory activity and to find out their influence in diabetic complications. Thus, Boswellia *serrata* Triana & Planch. (Burseraceae), *Lagerstroemia speciosa* (L.) Pers. (Lythraceae), *Ocimum gratissimum* (L.) (Lamiaceae) and *Syzygium cumin* (L.) Skeels. (Myrthaceae) and their respective major constituents, boswellic acid, corosolic acid, ursolic acid and ellagic acid, were studied for their inhibitory activity against rat lens AR, rat kidney AR, human recombinant AR. The results revealed that all the tested extracts and their active ingredients possess significant AR inhibitory actions in both *in vitro* and *in vivo* assays with urosolic acid showing the most potent effect (Ramarao *et al.,* 2012).

Methanolic as well as standardized extracts of *Andrographis paniculata* (Burm. f.) Wall. ex Nees (Acanthaceae) and its chief constituent, andrographolide, were studied using *in vitro* and *in vivo* methods. In the *in vitro* method, rat lens as well as kidney homogenates were used for the preparation of enzyme, whereas the effect of these test samples on the galactitol level in the eye lens was studied in a galactosemic rat model *in vivo*. The results of the study revealed that both extracts of the plant and its major compound, andrographolide, possess ARI activity *in vitro*. They were also found to significantly decrease galactitol accumulation *in vivo* (Veeresham *et al.,* 2012)

Four medicinal plant *(Morus alba* L., *Phyllanthus amarus* Schum. & Thonn., *Punica granatum* L., and *Stevia rebaudiana* Bertoni) standardized extracts and their major constituents (morusin, phyllanthin, punicalagin and stevioside) in the treatment of long-term diabetic complications by inhibition of aldose reductase (AR) enzyme. Rat lens and kidney homogenates, which contain rat lens AR (RLAR) and rat kidney AR (RKAR) crude enzymes, respectively, prepared in the laboratory and commercially available human recombinant AR (HRAR) were used to carry out *in vitro* bioassays. AR inhibitory activity was done by using ultraviolet-visible (UV-Vis). *In vivo* AR inhibitory activity, which involves determination of rat lens galactitol levels in galactosemic condition by using reverse phase high pressure liquid chromatography (RP-HPLC) and gas liquid chromatography (GLC) was determined. In the *in vitro* bioassays, punicalagin, the major constituent of *P. granatum* was found to have the most potent AR inhibitory activity with IC$_{50}$ values of 5.28, 6.22 and 4.70 µM in RLAR, RKAR, and HRAR assays, respectively, among the tested standardized extracts and pure compounds. The effect of punicalagin in suppressing rat lens galactitol levels in galactose-fed rat model was also superior to all other studied compounds including the positive control quercetin (Ramarao *et al.*, 2012).

The methanolic extract, standardized extract of flower and the major constituent butein were studied for their inhibitory activity against Rat Lens AR (RLAR), rat kidney AR; In addition, *in vivo* inhibition of lens galactitol accumulation in galactose-fed rat model was studied. The plant extracts and butein were shown to possess AR inhibitory activity in both *in vitro* and *in vivo* assays with equal potency to that of standard quercetin (Rajani *et al.*, 2015).

Ethanolic extracts of *Raphanus sativus* L. and their respective its organic solvent soluble fractions, including the ethyl acetate (EtOAc), *n* butanol (BuOH) and water layers, using DL-glyceraldehyde as a substrate, were studied for their inhibitory activity against rat lens AR, rat kidney AR. In addition, *in vivo* inhibition of lens galactitol accumulation by the major soluble fraction of the plant extract in galactose-fed rat model has been studied. The results show that all the tested soluble fraction of extracts possess significant AR inhibitory actions in both *in vitro* and *in vivo* assays with n-butanol showing the most the most potent effect (Ramarao *et al.*, 2012).

The AR inhibitory activities of the 24 Peruvian crude plant extracts were investigated; The AR inhibitory activities were evaluated using RLAR (Table 2.2). Only four crude extracts, Adiantum cf. *poiretii Wikstr.* (LNP-A9), *Gentianella tristicha* (Gilg) J.S. *Pringle* (LNP-P7), LNP-P83, and *Muehlenbeckia vulcanica* Meisn (LNP-P82), showed relatively high RLAR inhibition (over 50%) at 10 μg/mL. LNP-P83 showed significantly ($p < 0.05$) highest RLAR inhibition (87.55%) (Wang *et al.*, 2017).

Table 2.2 Rat lens aldose reductase inhibitory activities of 24 Peruvian infusion tea plant extracts from La Libertad. (Wang *et al.*, 2017).

S.No.	Species (Family)	Part used	Family	Comman name	%Inhibition (AR)
1.	Adiantum cf. poiretii Wikstr.	Aerial	Pteridaceae	Culantrillo	66.81±3.21m
2.	Malesherbia splendens Ricardi	Leaves+ flowers	Passifloraceae	Veronica	30.52 ±1.15k
3.	Gnaphalium dombeyanum DC./Achyrocline alata (Kunth) DC.	Aerial+flowers	Asteraceae	Arnica	16.67 ±0.85h
4.	Chuquiraga spinosa Less	Aerial	Asteraceae	Huamanpinta	13.21 ±0.71g
5.	Schkuhria pinnata (Lam.)Kuntze	Aerial	Asteraceae	Canchalagua	0 ± 0.01a
6.	Taraxacum officinale F.H. Wigg	Aerial /flowers	Asteraceae	Amargon	0 ± 0.009a
7.	Baccharis genistelloides (Lam.) Pers.	Leaves	Asteraceae	Karqueja	0 ± 0.01a
8.	Perezia multiflora (Bonpl.) Less.	Aerial	Asteraceae	Escorcioner, Corzonera	18.67 ± 0.93hi
9.	Senecio canescens (Bonpl.) Cuatrec.	Leaves	Asteraceae	Vira Vira	44.24 ± 2.21l
10.	Acanthoxanthium spinosum (L.)Fourr.	Aerial	Asteraceae	Juan Alonso, Amor seco	21.39 ± 1.07j
11.	Puya sp.	Aerial	Bromeliaceae	Hierba de Carnero	28.38 ± 0.92k
12.	Equisetum giganteum L.	Aerial	Equisetaceae	Cola de caballo	0.87 ± 0.03b
13.	Jatropha macrantha mull. Arg.	Roots	Euphorbiaceae	Huanarpo macho	5.51 ± 0.28e
14.	Desmodium molliculum (Kunth)DC.	Leaves	Fabaceae	Manayupa	12.86 ± 0.46g
15.	Otholobium pubescens (Poir.) J.W. Grimes	Aerial	Fabaceae	CulenBlanco	9.85 ± 0.54f
16.	Gentianella tristicha (Gilg) J.S.Pringle	Aerial	Gentianaceae	Hercampure	69.15 ± 4.54m

Table 2.2 Contd....

S.No.	Species (Family)	Part used	Family	Comman name	%Inhibition (AR)
17.	Ocimum basilicum L.	Aerial	Lamiaceae	Albahaca deolor	$16.55 \pm 0.83h$
18.	Lepechinia meyenii (Walp.) Epling	Aerial	Lamiaceae	salvia Paraguay	$44.43 \pm 2.22l$
19.	Buddleja americana L.	Flowers	Scrophulariaceae	Flor Blanca	$2.73 \pm 0.11c$
20.	Phoradendron sp	Leaves	Loranthaceae	Suelda con suelda	$87.55 \pm 3.74n$
21.	Huperzia crassa (Humb. & Bonpl. exWilld.) Rothm.	Leaves	Lycopodiaceae	Trensilla o enredadera	$19.58 \pm 0.98ij$
22.	Piper aduncum L.	Leaves	piperace	Matico	$30.41 \pm 1.58k$
23.	Cymbopogon citratus (DC.) Stapf.	Leaves	Poaceae	Hierba Luisa	$3.24 \pm 0.12d$
24.	Muehlenbeckia vulcanica Meisn.	Leaves	Polygonaceae	Mullaca	$65.92 \pm 3.30m$

References

Ángel Guzmán, Ricardo O. Guerrero. Inhibition of aldose reductase by herbs extracts and natural substances and their role in prevention of cataracts. REV CUBANA PLANT MED. 2005;10(3-4):1-7.

Chandrasekhar Akileshwari, Puppala Muthenna, Branislav Nastasijević, Gordana Joksić, J. Mark Petrash, Geereddy Bhanuprakash Reddy. Inhibition of Aldose Reductase by *Gentiana lutea* Extracts. Experimental Diabetes Research. 2012; doi:10.1155/2012/147965.

Halder N, Joshi S, Gupta SK. 2003. Lens aldose reductase inhibiting potential of some indigenous plants. *J Ethanopharmacol* 86: 113-116.

Hyun Ah Jung, M.D. Nurul Islam, Yong Soo Kwon, Seong Eun Jin, You Kyung Son, Jin Ju Park, Hee Sook Sohn, Jae Sue Choi. Extraction and identification of three major aldose reductase inhibitors from Artemisia Montana. Food and Chemical Toxicology. 2011; 49: 376–384.

Karasu C, Cumaoğlu A, Gürpinar AR, Kartal M, Kovacikova L, Milackova I, Stefek M. Aldose reductase inhibitory activity and antioxidant capacity of pomegranate extracts. 2012; Mar;5(1):15-20.

Kim J, Kim CS, Sohn E *et al.* 2011. KIOM-79 inhibits aldose reductase activity andcataractogenesis in Zucker diabetic fatty rats. *J Pharm Pharmacol* 63: 1301–1308.

Megha Saraswat, P Muthenna, P Suryanarayana, J Mark Petrash, G Bhanuprakash Reddy. Dietary sources of aldose reductase inhibitors: prospects for alleviating diabetic complications. Asia Pac J Clin Nutr. 2008; 17(4): 558-565.

Moghaddama MS, Anil Kumar P, Bhanuprakash RG, Ghole VS. Effect of Diabecon on sugar-induced lens opacity in organ culture: mechanism of action. *Journal of Ethnopharmacology* 2005; 97: 397–403.

Patel DK, Kumar R, Kumar M *et al.* 2012. Evaluation of *in vitro* aldose reductase inhibitory potential of different fraction of Hybanthus enneaspermus Linn F. Muell. *Asian Pac J Trop Biomed* 2: 134-139.

Po-Chow Hsieh, Guan-Jhong Huang, Yu-Ling Ho, Yaw-Huei Lin, Shyh-Shyun Huan, Ying-Chen Chiang, Mu-Chuan Tseng, Yuan-Shiun Chang. Activities of antioxidants, α-Glucosidase inhibitors and aldose reductase inhibitors of the aqueous extracts of four Flemingia species in Taiwan. Botanical Studies. 2010; 51: 293-302.

Rajani Garapelli,Ajmeera Rama Rao and Ciddi Veeresham (2015). Aldose reductase inhibitory activity of *Butea monosperma* for management of diabetic complications, Pharmacologia, 6(8):355-359.

Rajesh Kumar, Dinesh Kumar Patel, Damiki Laloo, Krishnamurthy Sairam, SivaHemalatha (2011). Inhibitory effect of two Indian medicinal plants on aldose reductase of rat lens *in vitro*. Asian Pacific Journal of Tropical Medicine. 4: 694-697.

Rama Rao Ajmeera, Veeresham Ciddi and Kaleab Asres, 2012. Potential of *Cassia auriculata* and *Saraca asoca s*tandardized extracts and their principle components for alleviating diabetic complications. International journal phytomedicine 4(4); 558-563.

Rama Rao Ajmeera, Veeresham Ciddi and Kaleab Asres. 2012. *In vitro* and *in vivo* inhibitory activity of four Indian medicinal plant extracts and their major components on rat aldose reductase and generation of advance glycation endproducts. Phytotherapy Research. DOI:10.1002/ptr.4786.

RN Gacche, NA Dhole. Aldose reductase inhibitory, anti-cataract and antioxidant potential of selected medicinal plants from the Marathwada region, India. Natural Product Research 2011a; 25(7): 760–763.

RN Gacche, NA Dhole. Profile of aldose reductase inhibition, anti-cataract and free radical scavenging activity of selected medicinal plants: An attempt to standardize the botanicals for amelioration of diabetes complications. Food and Chemical Toxicology. 2011b; 49: 1806–1813.

Sri Fatmawati, Kenji Kurashiki, Sayaka Takeno, Yongung Kim, Kuniyoshi Shimizu, Masao Sato, Katsumi Imaizumi, Kaori Takahashi, Shinji Kamiya, Shuhei Kaneko, Ryuichiro Kondo. The Inhibitory Effect on Aldose Reductase by an Extract of *Ganoderma lucidum*. Phytother. Res. 2009; 23: 28–32.

Suryanarayana P, P Anil Kumar, Megha Saraswat, J Mark Petrash, G Bhanuprakash Reddy. Inhibition of aldose reductase by tannoid principles of Emblica officinalis: implications for the prevention of sugar cataract.Molecular vision. 2004; 10:148-54.

Termentzi A, P Alexiou, V J Demopoulos, E Kokkalou. The aldose reductase inhibitory capacity of Sorbus domestica fruit extracts depends on their phenolic content and may be useful for the control of diabetic complications. Pharmazie. 2008; 63: 693–696.

Veeresham C, Swetha E Rama Rao A, and Kaleab A. 2012. Aldose reductase inhibitory activity of standardized extracts and the major constituents of *Andrographis paniculata*. Phytotherapy Research. DOI:10.1002/ptr.4722.

Xu Z, Yang H, Zhou M *et al.* 2010. Inhibitory effect of total lignan from *Fructus Arctii* on aldose reductase. *Phytother Res* 24: 472–473.

Young-Shin Chung, Yun-Hee Choi, Seok-Jong Lee, Sun a Choi, Jang-ha Lee, Harriet Kim, Eun-Kyung Hong. Water extract of *Aralia elata* prevents cataractogenesis *in vitro* and *in vivo*. *Journal of Ethnopharmacology* 2005; 101: 49–54.

Zhiqiang Wang, Seung Hwan Hwang, Yanymee N. Guillen Quispe, Paul H. Gonzales Arce,Soon Sung Lim. Investigation of the antioxidant and aldose reductase inhibitory activities of extracts from Peruvian tea plant infusions. Food Chemistry 231 (2017) 222–230.

Chapter 3

Plants as Antiglycation Agents: Nutraceuticals for the Management of Diabetic Complications

3.1 Introduction

The formation of AGEs may alter the physicochemical properties of the proteins, and in turn adversely affect their functional properties (Monnier *et al.*, 2005). Previous studies have established the role of AGEs in the development of diabetic complications (Singh *et al.*, 2001; Ahmed, 2005; Daroux *et al.*, 2010). Therefore, the mitigation of protein glycation will be an effective medium of preventing or ameliorating these complications. There is a continuous demand for agents with antiglycation properties, as they may be useful in preventing diabetic complications (Rahbar *et al.*, 2003; Jagtap and Patil, 2010). Though some synthetic antiglycation agents like aminoguanidine and pyridoxamine have been discovered, they have serious toxicity issues (Peng *et al.*, 2011). Therefore, food-derived antiglycation agents will be more appropriate in the management of diabetic complications due to their safety and availability to the general populace.

Approach for Detection of AGEs

Structures of various AGEs have been elucidated and the role of AGEs in diseases like diabetes has been clarified, study of glycated proteins has attracted more interest. However, the studies involving early and advanced glycation products are still suffering owing to the lack of a gold standard technique for their detection and measurement (Jalaluddin *et al.*, 2015). A summary of the advantages and disadvantages associated with the major techniques used for the detection of AGEs is provided in Table 3.1.

Table 3.1 Merits and demerits of major techniques used for the measurement of AGEs. (Jalaluddin *et al.,* 2015).

Technique	Merits	Demerits
Immunohistochemistry	Tissue localization of AGEs can be determined, and its colocalization with RAGEs can also be determined.	Lack sensitivity and reproducibility
ELISA	Rapid and currently most frequently used.	Specificity of antibodies is often difficult to characterize and due to steric constraints, all epitopes are not accessible to the antibodies.
HPLC	Provides very precise quantification of AGEs.	Cumbersome chromatographic systems and long retention time
LC/MS	Most accurate technique	Very expensive
UV–Visible spectroscopy	A quick preliminary tool for initial monitoring of glycation reaction	Not appropriate for quantitative estimation of glycation products
Fluorescence spectroscopy	Most valuable, simple and most commonly used methods for the measurement of AGEs	Nonfluorescent AGEs cannot be determined
Boronate affinity chromatography	Simple and efficient	Nonspecific interactions between boronate and nonglycosylated proteins
Fluorescent phenylboronate gel electrophoresis	A simple, cost-effective detection and analysis tool for glycated proteins and provides direct visualization of glycated proteins	Only suitable for the analysis of samples with limited complexity

This book is an attempt to compile a repository of plant extracts and phyto constituents, which have been validated to display antiglycation potential *in vitro* and *in vivo* (chemical structures shown in figure 3.1). This will serve as a guide to future references for researchers and pharmaceutical industries, for further studies aimed at isolation of their active components and large-scale production. It will also assist diabetics and their families in the choice of foods that will be consumed, in order to ameliorate the debilitating effects of diabetes and its complications. Promising results were obtained in many of the studies reported in this chapter, only few studies gave detailed characterization of the active compounds responsible for the antiglycation activities. In order to give detailed description of the antiglycation potentials of these foods, the plants are presented on the basis of their Extracts, fractions and compounds from medicinal plants.

Figure 3.1 Structures of Phyto chemical isolated from plant extracts with antiglycation potential.

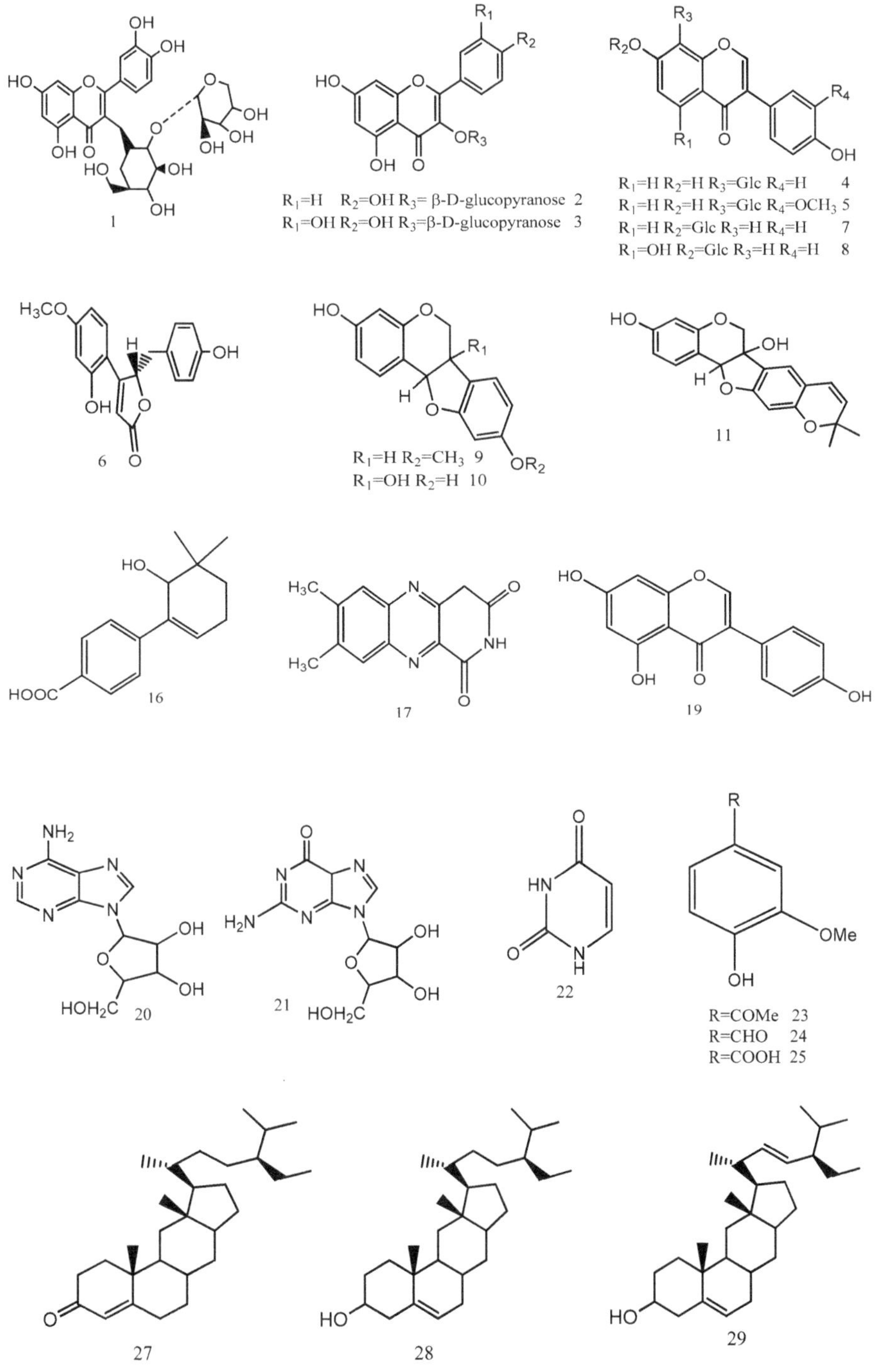
1
R_1=H R_2=OH R_3= β-D-glucopyranose 2
R_1=OH R_2=OH R_3=β-D-glucopyranose 3
R_1=H R_2=H R_3=Glc R_4=H 4
R_1=H R_2=H R_3=Glc R_4=OCH_3 5
R_1=H R_2=Glc R_3=H R_4=H 7
R_1=OH R_2=Glc R_3=H R_4=H 8
6
R_1=H R_2=CH_3 9
R_1=OH R_2=H 10
11
16
17
19
20
21
22
R=COMe 23
R=CHO 24
R=COOH 25
27
28
29

Figure 3.1 *Contd....*

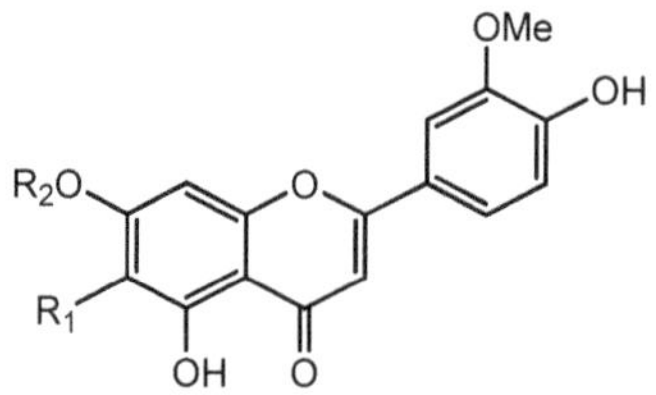

R$_1$=R$_2$=H   18
R$_1$= β-boivinose, R$_2$=β-Glucose   32
R$_1$= β–(L)-boivinose, R$_2$=H   33
R$_1$= β–fucose, R$_2$=H   34
R$_1$= α–rhamnose(1-2)β–fucose, R$_2$=H   35

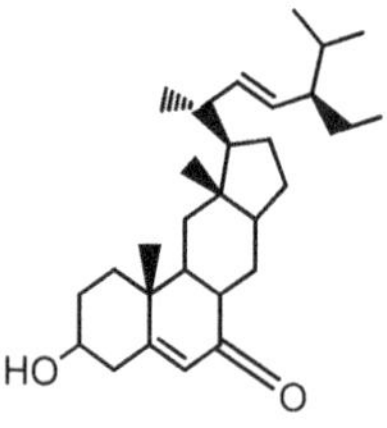

30

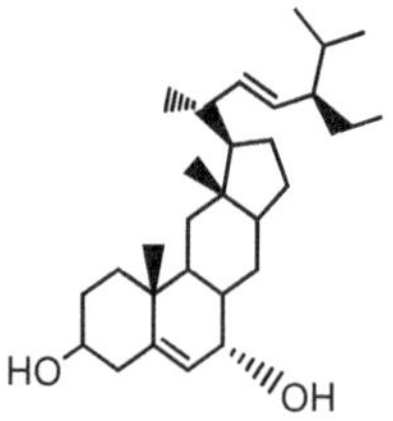

31

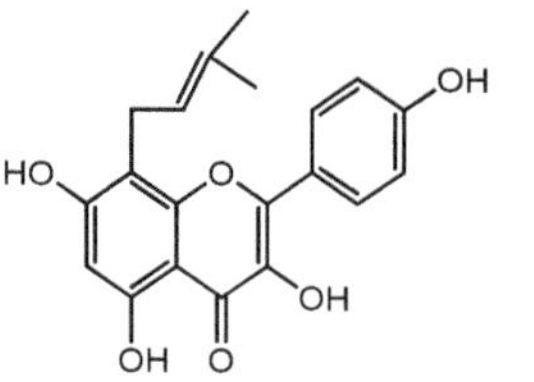

32

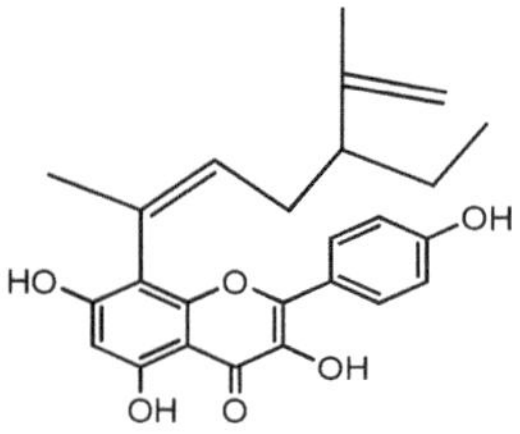

33

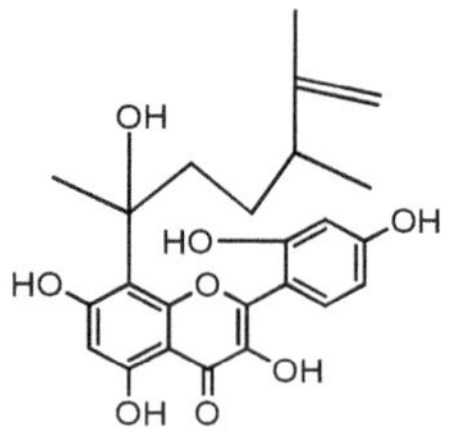

34

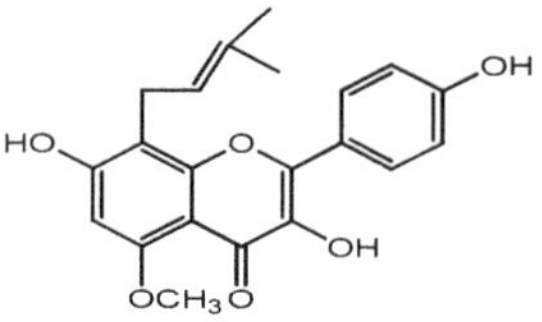

35

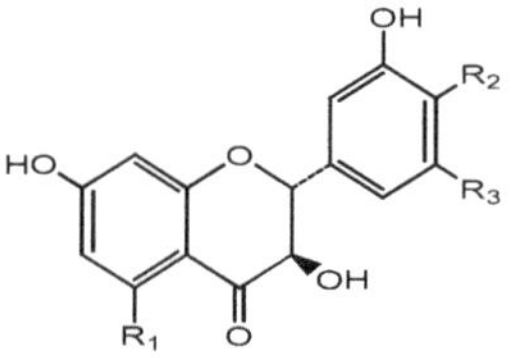

R$_1$=H R$_2$=OH R$_3$=H (36)
R$_1$=OH R$_2$=H R$_3$=OH (37)

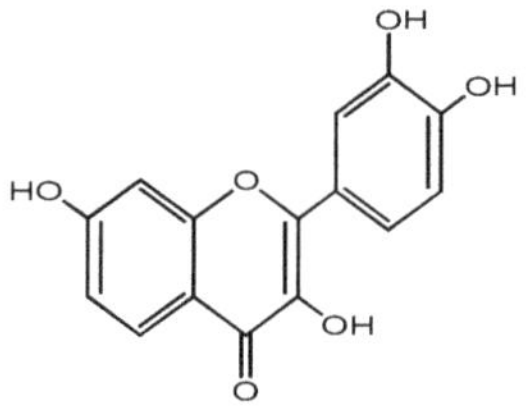

38

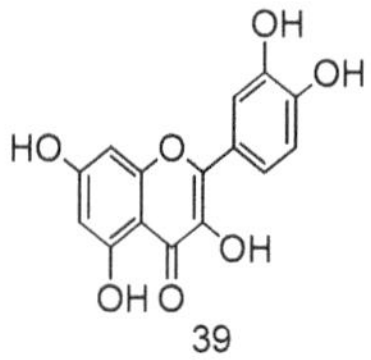

39

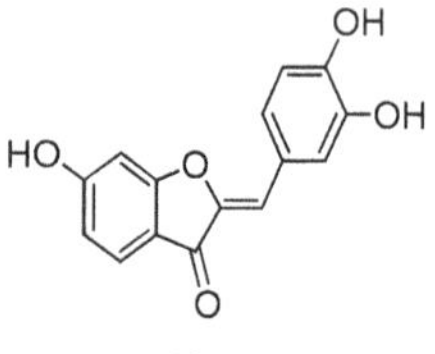

40

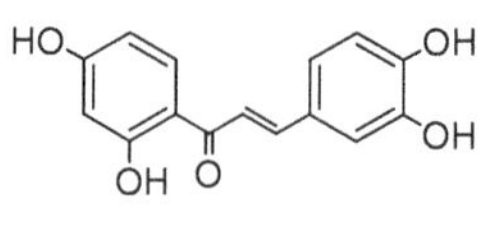

41

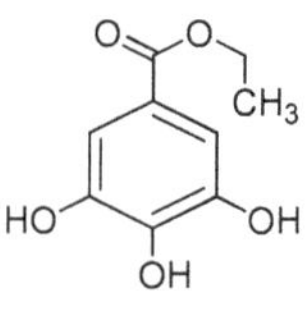

42

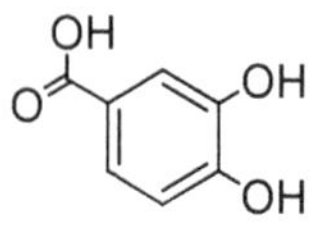

43

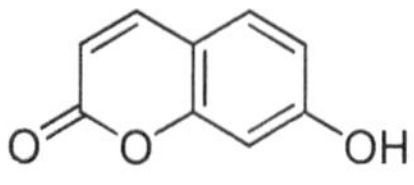

44

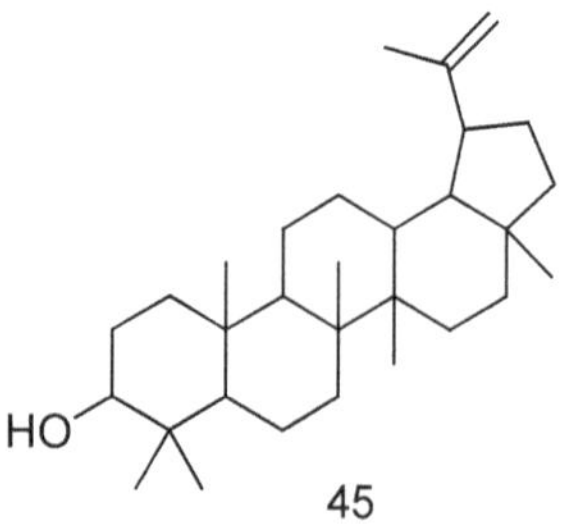

45

Figure 3.1 *Contd....*

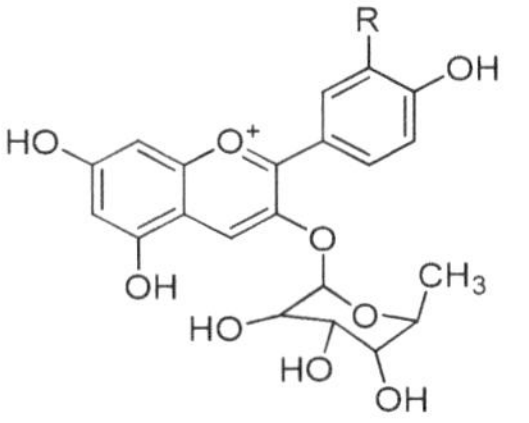

R=OH 46
R=H 47

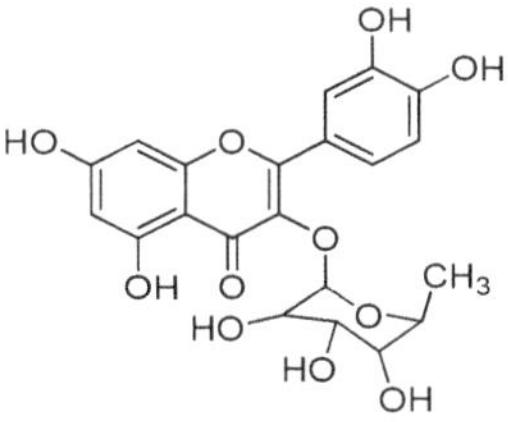

48

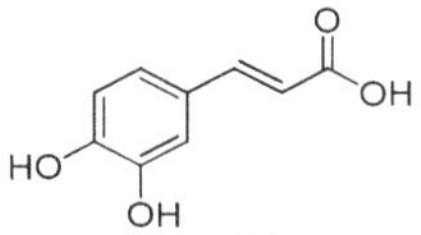

49

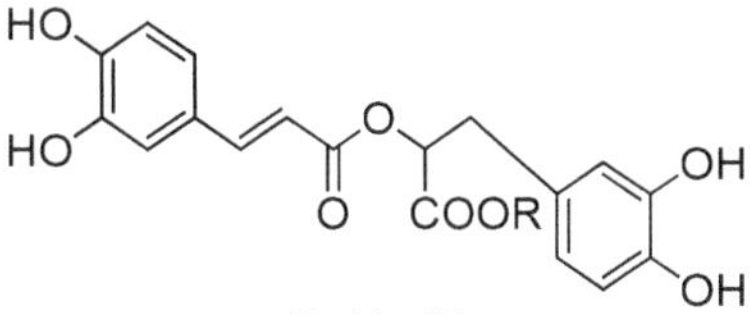

R=Me 50
R=H 51

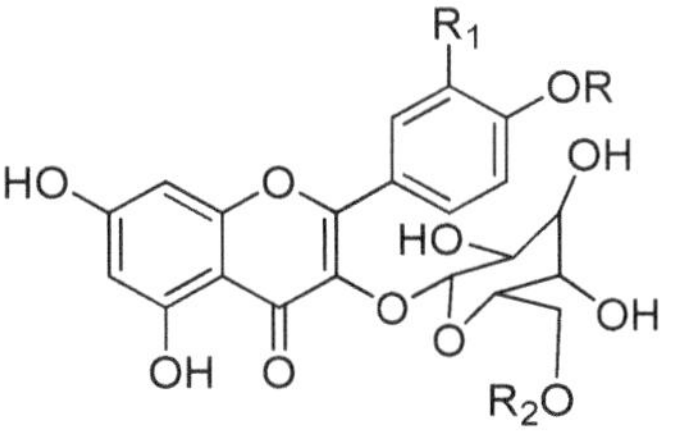

R=Me	R_1=H	R_2=H		52
R=H	R_1=H	R_2=H		53
R=H	R_1=OH	R_2=H		54
R=Me	R_1=H	R_2=Rhamnosyl		55
R=H	R_1=H	R_2=Rhamnosyl		56

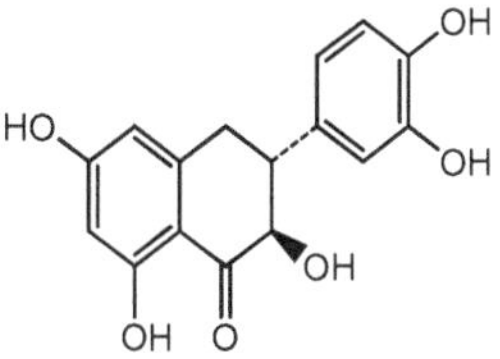

57

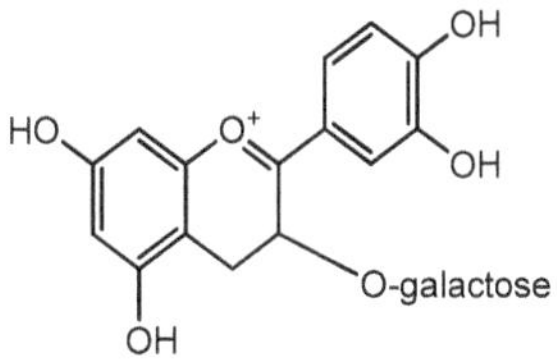

58

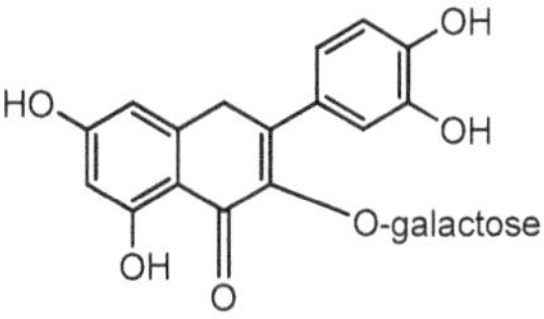

59

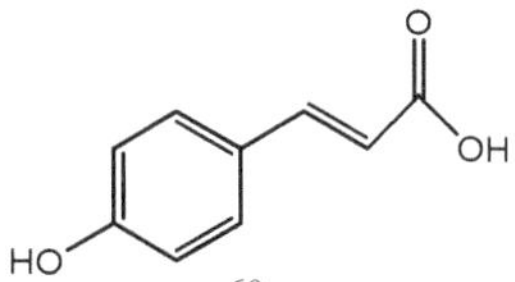

60

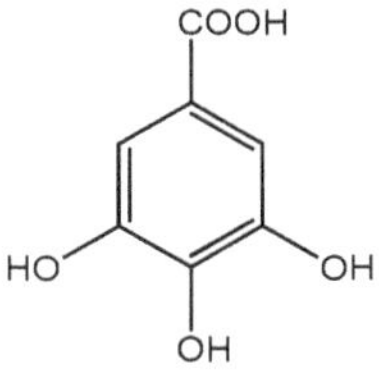

61

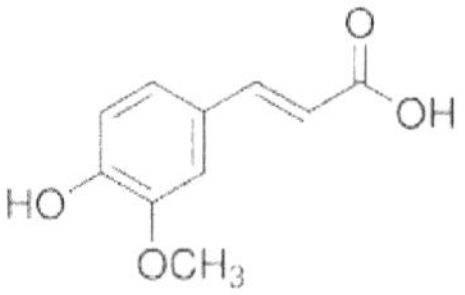

62

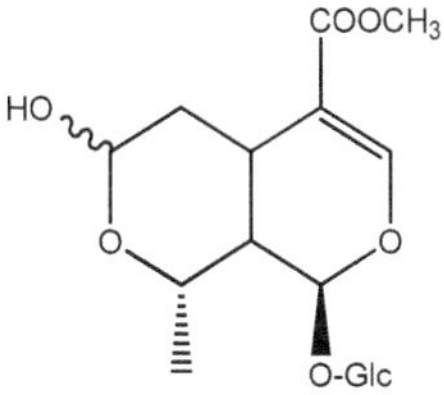

63

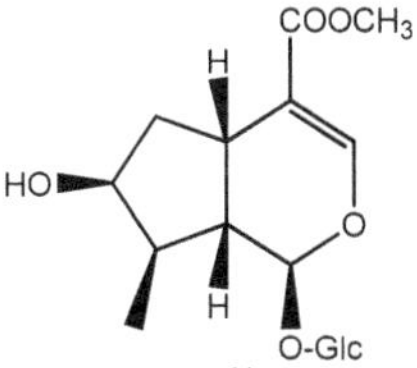

64

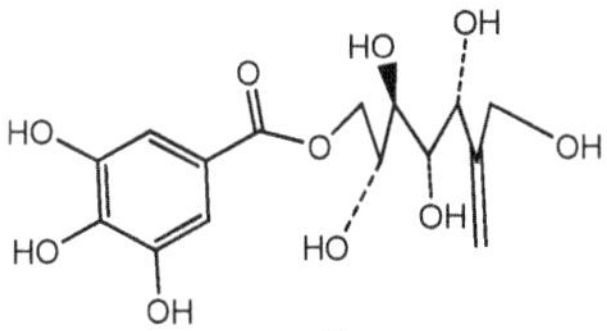

65

Figure 3.1 *Contd....*

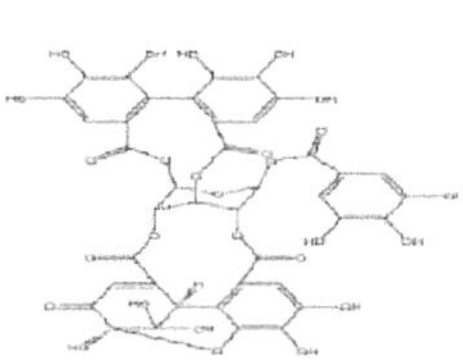

66

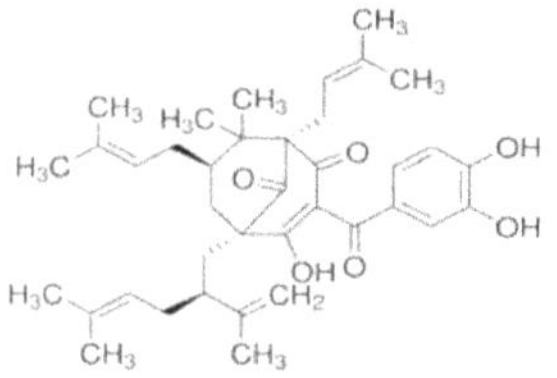

67

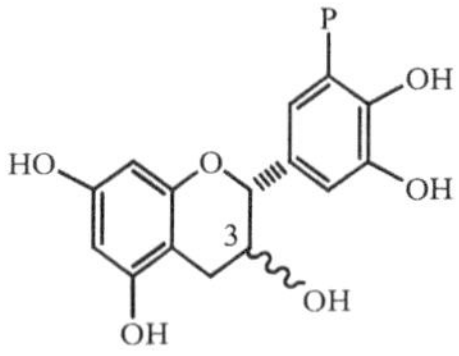

P=OH 3β   68
P=OH 3α   69
P=H   3β   70
P=H   3α   71

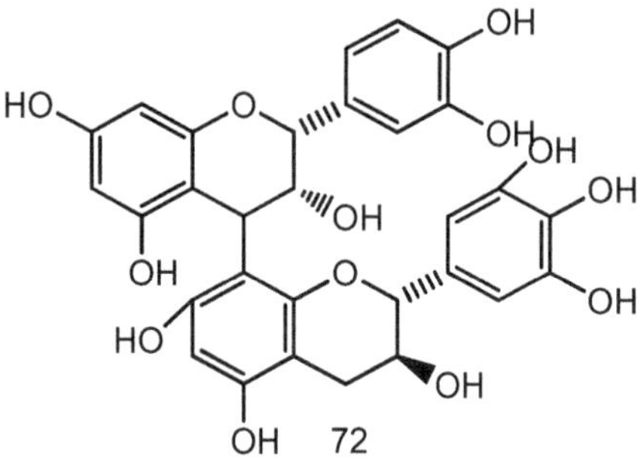

72

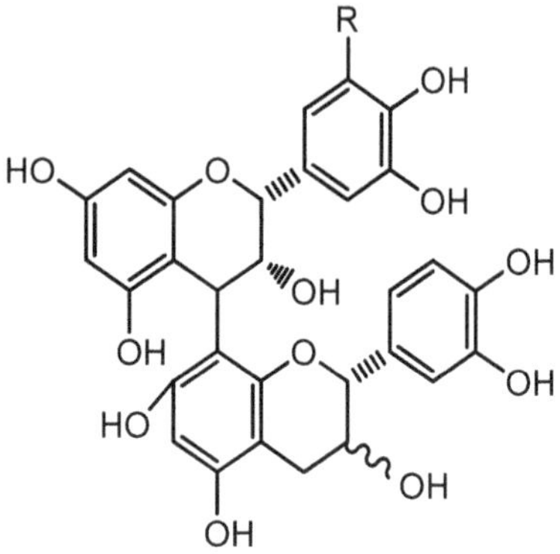

R=OH   73
R=H   74

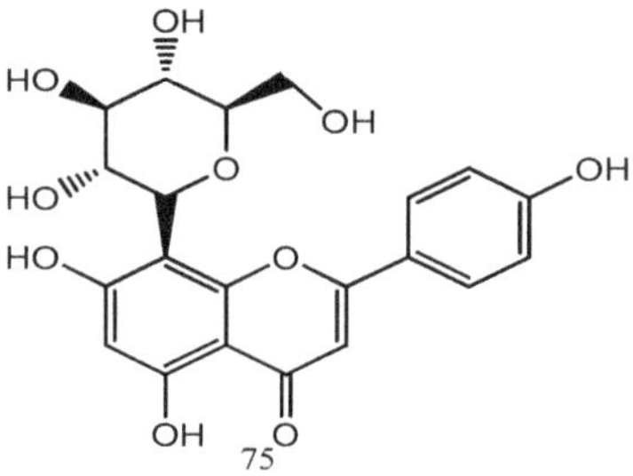

75

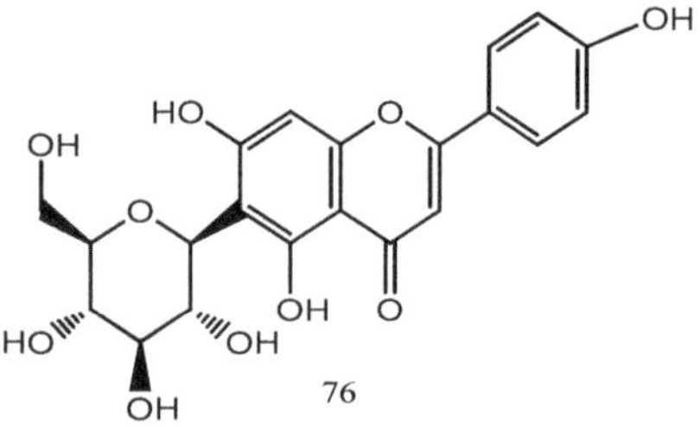

76

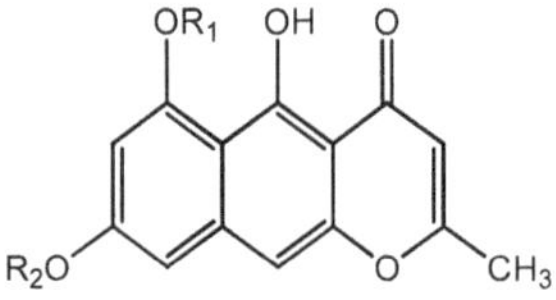

R₁=glucosyl R₂=H   77
R₁=gentibiosyl R₂=CH₃ 78

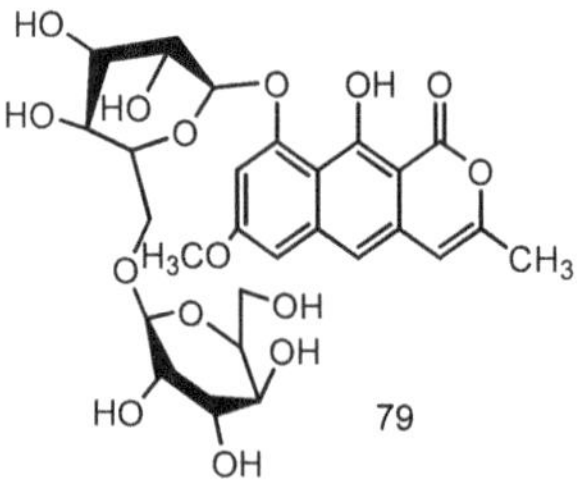

79

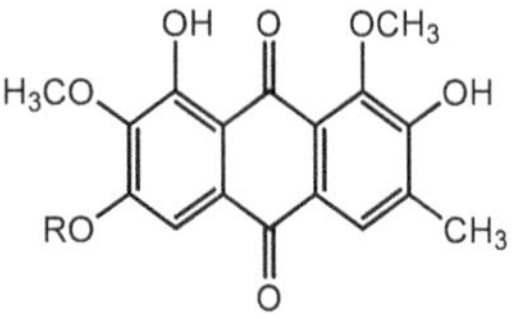

R=H   80
R=CH₃ 81

Figure 3.1 *Contd….*

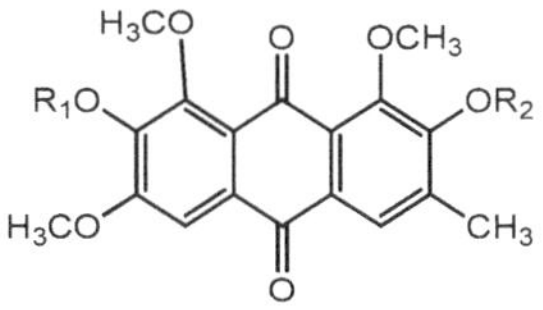

R₁=R₂=H 82
R₁=H R₂=glc 83

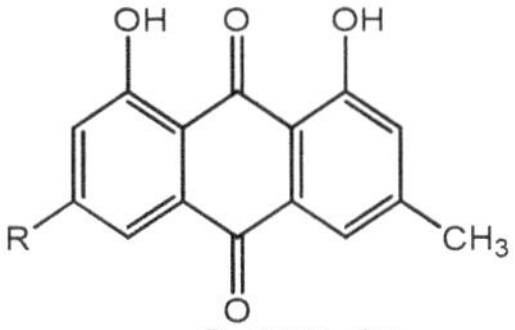

R=OCH₃ 84
R=OH 85
R=H 86

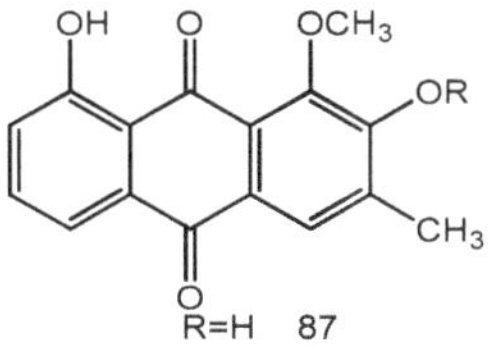

R=H 87
R=glc 88

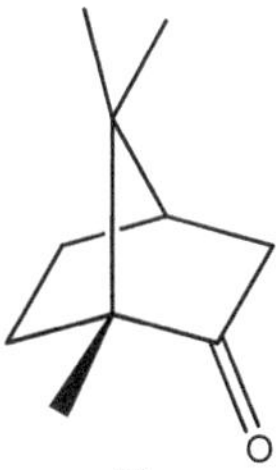

89

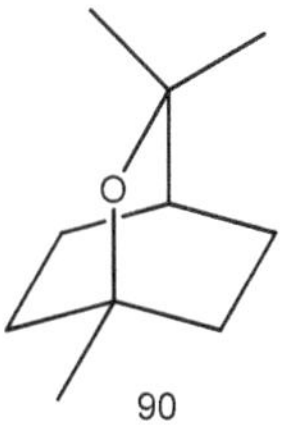

90

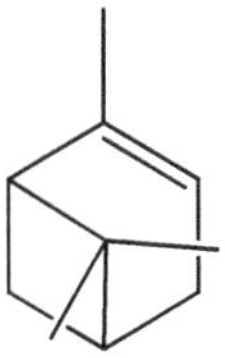

91

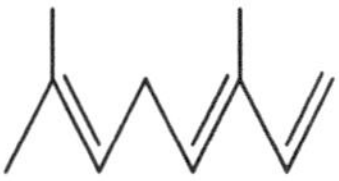

92

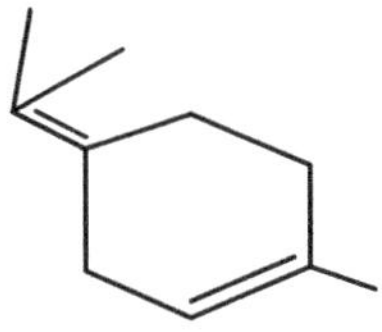

93

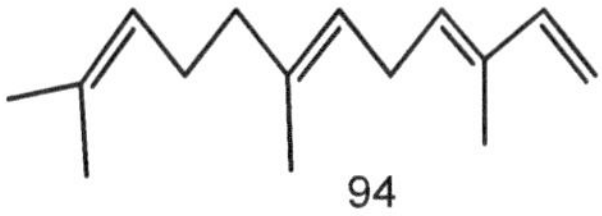

94

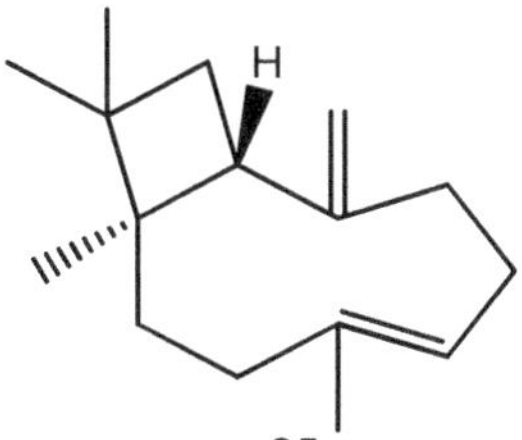

95

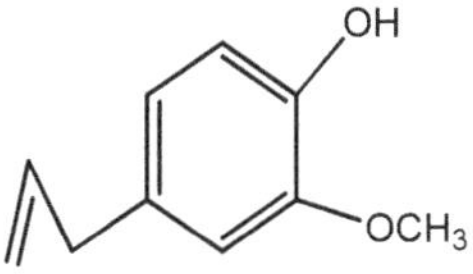

96

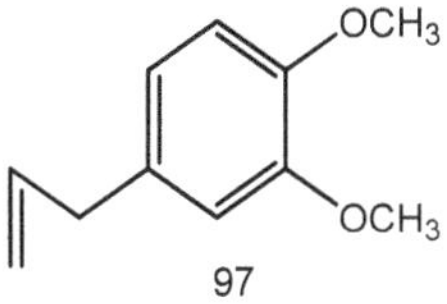

97

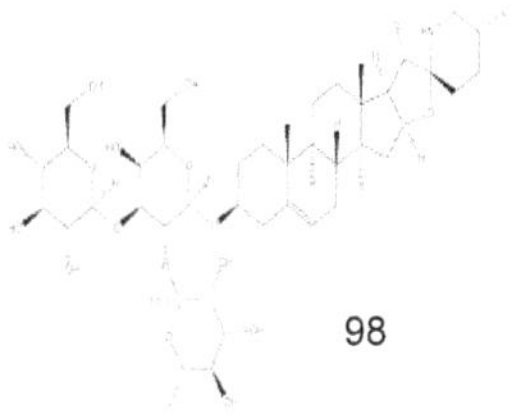

98

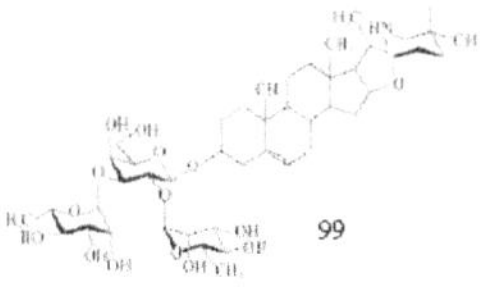

99

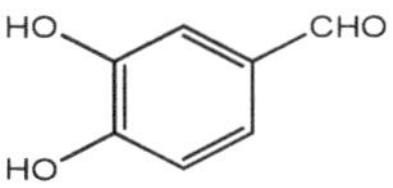

100

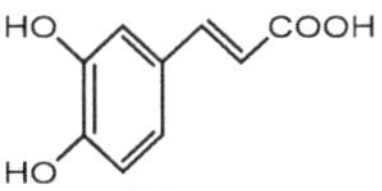

101

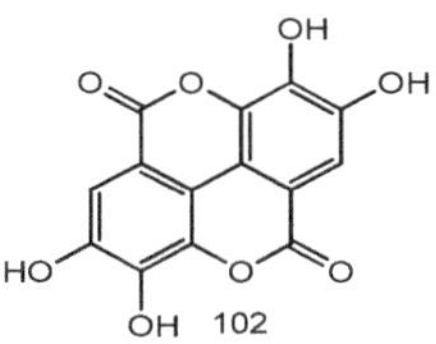

102

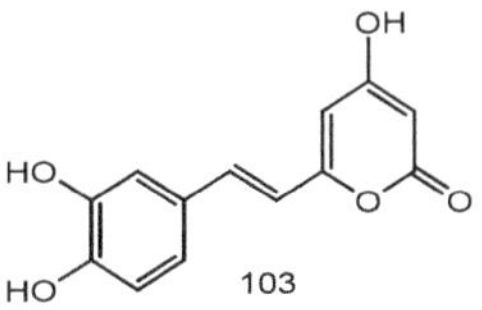

103

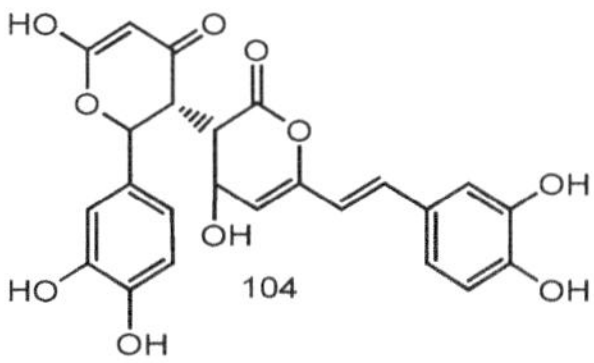

104

Figure 3.1 *Contd….*

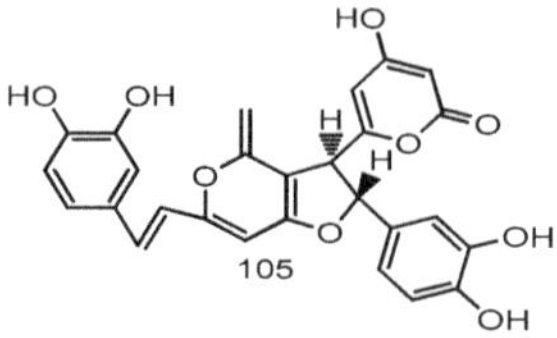

105
106
107
108
109
110
R1=H R2=Xyl R3=Rha   111
R1=Me R2=Glc R3=Rha   112
R1=Me R2=Xyl R3=Rha   113
R1=H R2=H   R3=Rha   116
R1=Me R2=H   R3=Rha   117
R1=H R2=H   R3=H   118
R=Glc 114
R=H   115
119
120
121
122
123
124
125

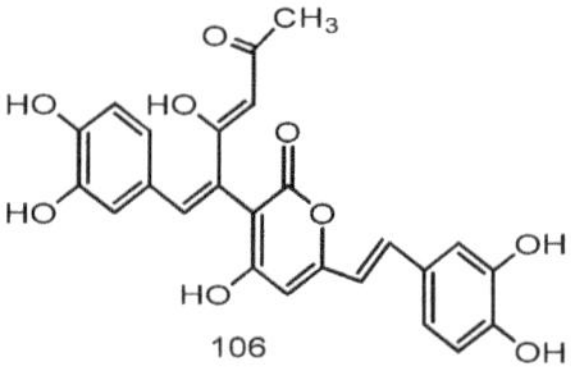

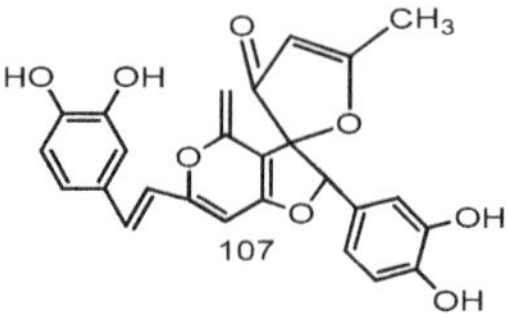

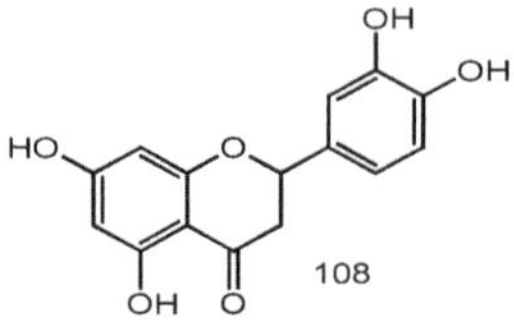

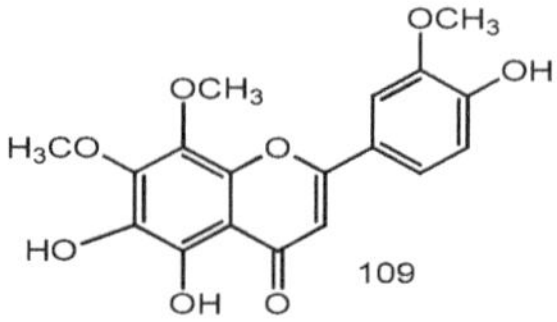

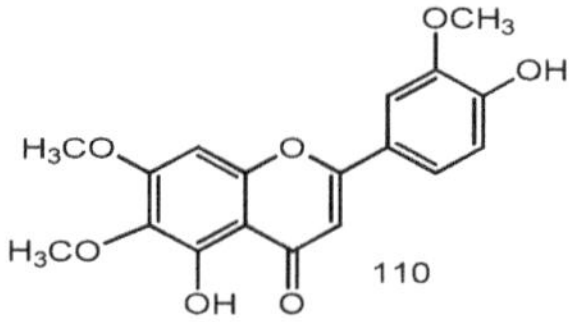

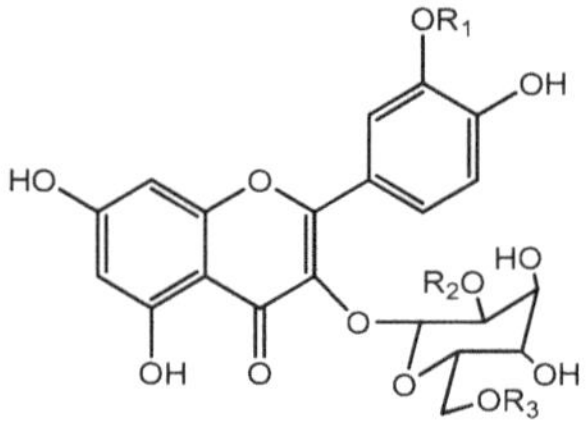

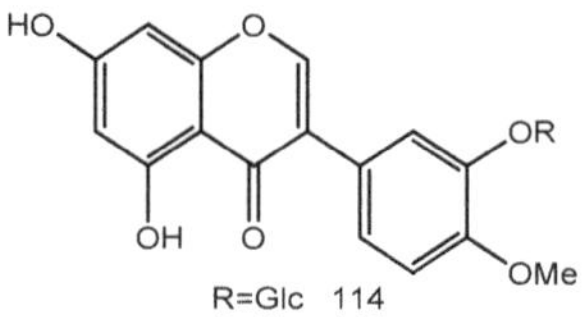

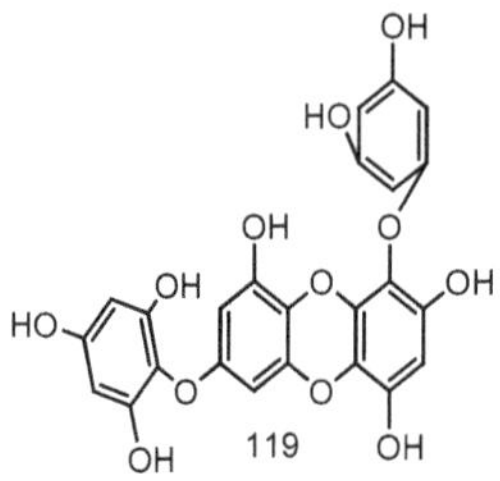

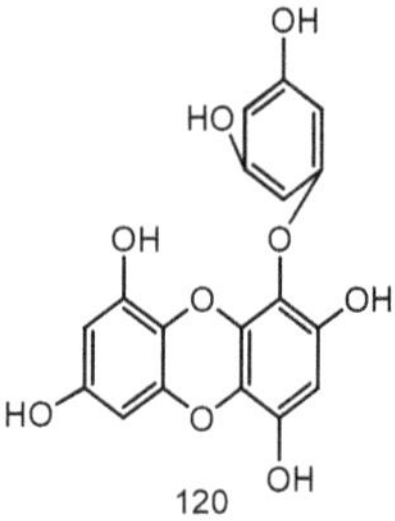

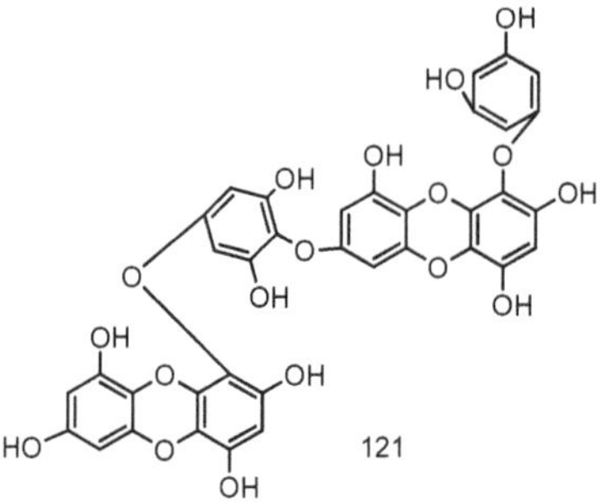

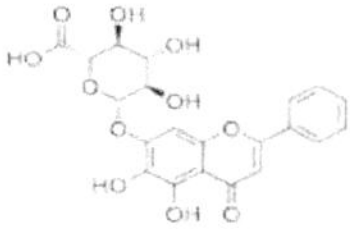

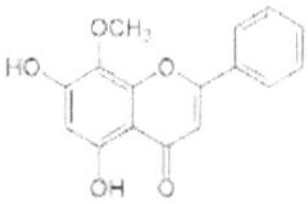

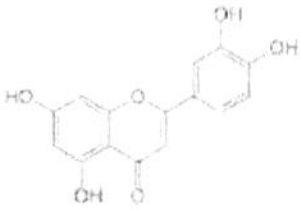

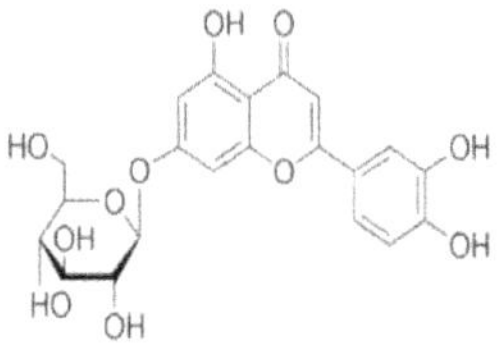

Extracts, fractions and compounds from medicinal plants:

Extracts of two flavonoid-rich South American herbs, *Achyrocline satureoides* and *Ilex paraguariensis,* showed strong abilities to prevent the glycation of proteins induced by dicarbonyls at a 1/100 dilution of the herbal infusions, which were comparable to the inhibitory effects of millimolar amounts of aminoguanidine and carnosine as well as micromolar amounts of ascorbic acid (Gugliucci and Menini, 2002).

Antiglycation activity of aqueous ethanolic extracts from 25 plant tissues collected in Korea were determined and the few most effective ones in descending order were: *Allium cepa* (skin), *Lllicium religiosum* (bark and wood), *Fagopyrum esculentum* (hull), and *Origanum officinalis* (leaf). IC_{50} values of extracts effects on Fluorescence Formation in the BSA-Fructose Reaction *in vitro* shown in table 3.2. Meanwhile, aged garlic extract was suggested as a potential inhibitor for AGEs (Imai *et al.,* 1994; Kim and Kim, 2003; Ahmad *et al.,* 2006).

Table 3.2 Effects of Plant Extracts on Fluorescence Formation in the BSA-Fructose Reaction *in Vitro*. (Kim and Kim, 2003)

S.No.	Species	Part used	Family	IC_{50} (µg/mL)
1.	*Allium cepa*	skin	Liliaceae	16.8 ± 5.0s
2.	*Illicium religiosum*	bark	Magnoliaceae	25.6 ± 4.7rs
3.	*Fagopyrum esculentum*	hull	Polygonaceae	39.0 ± 3.02q
4.	*Origanum officinalis*	leaf	Labiatae	41.4 ± 1.74pq
5.	*Illicium religiosum*	wood	Magnoliaceae	46.5±4.80opq
6.	*Rosmarinus officinalis*	leaf	Labiatae	48.5±0.35opq
7.	*Pyrus pyrifolia*	bark	Rosaceae	49.6 ±16.5nop
8.	*Acanthopanax senticosus*	bark	Araliaceae	50.8 ± 3.4no
9.	*Eugenia caryophllata*	leaf	Myrtaceae	55.9 ± 0.54mn
10.	*Erigeron annuus*	whole	Compositae	56.6 ± 6.5mn
11.	*Paeonia suffruticosa*	root	Ranunculaceae	63.9 ± 0.8lm
12.	*Thymus vulgaris*	leaf	*Labiatae*	85.0 ± 13.9k
13.	*Oryza sativa* var.	Suwon	Gramineae	92.5 ± 3.2jk
14.	*Paeonia lactiflora*	root	Paeoniaceae	94.5 ± 3.2j
15.	*Camellia sinensis*	leaf	Theaceae	97.9 ± 18.9ij
16.	*Laurus nobilis*	leaf	Lauraceae	105 ± 8.19hi
17.	*Eucommia ulmoides*	leaf	Eucomimiaceae	109.7 ± 2.5h
18.	*Euonymus alata*	root	Celastraceae	118.9 ± 1.4g
19.	*Cornus officinalis*	fruit	Cornaceae	158.0 ± 10.9ef
20.	*Phellodendron amjrense*	leaf	Rutaceae	160.0 ± 0.8ef
21.	*Torreya nucifera*	leaf	Taxaceae	166.1 ± 0.8de
22.	*Thuja orientalis*	leaf	Cypressaceae	170.0 ± 2.0d
23.	*Saururus chinensis*	leaf	Saururaceae	174.5 ± 8.1cd
24.	*Cinamomum cassia*	bark	Lauraceae	182.7 ± 10.1c
25.	*Schizandra chinensis*	fruit	Magnoliaceae	352.4 ± 2.5a
	Aminoguanidine			27.7 ± 3.2r

Yoshikawa *et al.,* 2003 reported that, the aqueous methanolic extracts from different *Salacia* Species (*S. chinensis, S. oblonga* and *S. Reticulata*) evaluated their inhibitory activity on AGEs. The methanol extract from stems of *Salacia* Species was found to possess a strong inhibitory effect on the formation of Amadori compounds and AGEs. Among them, *S. chinensis,* extract was show high inhibitory glycation with IC_{50} value 139 (mg/mL) (Yoshikawa *et al.,* 2003).

Kim *et al.,* 2004 reported that, the flavanol glycoside, quercetin 3-O-α-L-arabinopyranosyl-(1->2)-β-D-glucopyranoside (1), and known flavanols kaempferol 3-O-β-D-glucopyranoside (astragalin) (2), quercetin 3-O-β-D-glucopyranoside (isoquercitrin) (3) were isolated from the 50% ethanolic extract of leaves of *Eucommia ulmoides.* These compounds exhibited potent glycation inhibitory activity comparable to that of aminoguanidine, a known glycation inhibitor.

Aqueous extracts of *Toona sinensis* Roem. (Meliaceae) and *Graptopetalum paragugayene* E. Walther (Crassulaceae) were reported to prevent the formation of AGEs from low density lipoprotein (LDL) glycation induced by glucose and glyoxal (Hsieh *et al.,* 2005).

Kang *et al.,* 2006 reported that, the effect of sun ginseng (SG, heat-processed *Panax ginseng* C. A. MEYER at 120 °C) on the renal AGEs level in diabetic control rats was significantly higher than in normal rats, but it was effectively lowered by SG administrations to an almost normal level. It declined from 0.96 to 0.81 and 0.80 arbitrary units (AU) by the administration of 50 or 100 mg/kg body weight/day of SG, respectively.

Five crude drug constituents of Wen-Pi-Tang (*Rhei Rhizoma, Ginseng* Radix, Aconiti Tuber, Zingiberis Rhizoma and Glycyrrhizae Radix), and a Chinese medical prescription to treat moderate renal failure, were chosen to examine their capability to prevent protein glycation. *Rhei Rhizoma* displayed the most potent activity, *Zingiberis Rhizoma* and *Glycyrrhizae* radix showed relatively moderate activity and Aconiti Tuber and Ginseng Radix presented weak activity (Nakagawa *et al.,* 2005). Meanwhile, compounds like tannins, especially rhatannin, RG-tannin and procyanidin B-2 3,3´-di-*O*-gallate obtained from *Rhei Rhizoma* and *Glycyrrhizae radix* exerted superior activities that were stronger than the positive control aminoguanidine. The isolated flavones such as licochalcone A and licochalcone B, and anthraquinones such as emodin and aloe-emodin, also showed obvious inhibitory activity against glycation (Yokozawa *et al.,* 2006).

Jakyakgamcho-tang (JGT) is a well-known traditional herbal formula, which consists of the radix of *Paeonia lactiflora* Pallas (PR) and the radix and rhizome of *Glycyrrhiza uralensis* Fisch (GR). Study was to evaluate the inhibitory and breaking activities of JGT, PR, and GR against AGEs. GT, PR, and GR extracts were prepared in hot water. In the *in vitro* AGE formation assay, JGT and PR dose-dependently inhibited AGE-BSA formation (half-maximal inhibitory concentration, IC_{50}, = 41.41 ± 0.36 and 6.84 ± 0.09 μg/mL, respectively). In the breakdown assay of the preformed AGE-BSA-collagen complexes, JGT and PR exhibited potent breaking activities (IC_{50} = 6.72 ± 1.86 and 7.45 ± 0.47 μg/mL, respectively). However, GR showed a weaker inhibitory activity and no breaking activity against AGEs (Kim *et al.*, 2016).

Two isoflavone C-glucosides, puerarin (4), PG-3 (5), a but-2-enolide, (±)-puerol B (6), two isoflavone O-glucosides, daidzin (7) and genistin (8), and three pterocarpans, (-)-medicarpin (9), (-)-glycinol (10) and (-)-tuberosin (11), were isolated from a MeOH extract of the roots of *Pueraria lobata*, were evaluated for their inhibitory activity on AGEs formation *in vitro*. Among the tested compound, puerarin (4), PG-3 (5), and (±)-puerol B (6) exhibited more potent inhibitory activity than the positive control aminoguanidine (Kim *et al.*, 2006).

In another study, a new 2-arylbenzofuran, puerariafuran (12), as well as three known compounds, coumestrol (13), daidzein (14), and genistein (15), were isolated from a MeOH extract of the roots of *Pueraria lobata* and assed the inhibitory effects on AGE formation. Among the tested compound, puerariafuran and coumestrol exhibited a superior inhibitory activity against AGEs formation with IC_{50}values of 0.53 and 0.19μM, respectively (Jang *et al.*, 2006).

A new sesquiterpenoid 1(16) along with flavonoids: chrysoeriol (18), genistein (19), (chrysoeriol 6-*C*-β-boivinopyranosyl-7-*O*-β-glucopyranoside) (32), (alternanthin) 33, (chrysoeriol 6-*C*-β-fucopyranoside) 34, and chrysoriol 6-*C*-α-rhamnopyranosyl-(1→2)-β-fucopyranoside 35; Sterols: stigmast-4-en-3-one (27), β-sitosterol (28), stigmasterol (29), stigmastanone (30), and 7a-hydroxysitosterol (31); *N*-containing compounds: lumichrome (2), adenosine (20), guanosine (21), uracil (22), 6-methoxy-benzoxazolinone (26) and vanillin derivatives: acetovanillone (23), vanillin (24) vanillic acid (25), were isolated from the style of *Zea mays* L. and carried out the their anti-glycation activity and % inhibition is summarized in table 3. Among, the tested compounds alternanthin (33), chrysoeriol 6-*C*-β –fucopyranoside (34), and genistein (19) inhibited glycation, but none of the isolated sterols affected glycation of the *N*-containing compounds, only guanosine (21) inhibited glycation. Vanillin (24), which possesses an aldehyde group and its derivatives, did not exhibit inhibitory activity (Suzuki *et al.*, 2007).

Two dihydro flavanol glycosides, engeletin and astilbin, were isolated from an EtOAc extract of the leaves of *Stelechocarpus cauliflorus* R.E. Fr. (Annonaceae), whose root is used for the treatment of stomach aches. Astilbin was more potent than engeletin to prevent the formation of AGEs, and was about as potent as a reported natural inhibitor quercetin (Wirasathien et al., 2007).

Table 3.3 % Inhibitory activities values of isolated from the style of *Zea mays* L against AGEs (Suzuki *et al.,* 2007)

Compounds	% Inhibition
Chrysoeriol (18)	----
Genistein (19),	95
Acetovanillone (23),	-------
Vanillin (24)	28
Vanillic Acid (25),	-----
(Chrysoeriol 6-*C*-B -Boivinopyranosyl-7-*O*-B - Glucopyranoside) 32,	12
(Alternanthin) 33,	69
(Chrysoeriol 6-*C*-B -Fucopyranoside) 34,	81
Chrysoriol 6-*C*-A-Rhamnopyranosyl-(1→2)-B- Fucopyranoside 35;	2
And Sterols: Stigmast-4-En-3-One (27),	-----
B-Sitosterol (28),	-----
Stigmasterol (29),	------
Stigmastanone (30),	------
N-Containing Compounds: Lumichrome (17),	-----
Adenosine (20),	20
6-Methoxy-Benzoxazolinone (26)	41
Uracil (22),	5
Guanosine (21),	63
New Sesquiterpenoid 1(16)	2
7α-Hydroxysitosterol (31);	------
Amino Guanidine(10mm)	57.1

Three prenylated flavanols and one prenylated flavanone isolated from the root extract of *Sophora flavescens* and examined for their AGEs inhibitory activities (Jung *et al.,* 2008b). The results summarized in Table 3.3 indicated that all of the prenylated flavanols, flavanone isolated from the active methylene dichloride and ethyl acetate fractions show varying degrees of activity on AGEs formation. prenylated flavanols 1–3 and the prenylated flavanone 11 possessed good inhibitory activities against AGE formation compared with the standard aminoguanidine (Table 3.4). All active prenylated flavonoids have a hydroxyl group at the 3 position, indicating that the 3-hydroxyl group may be one of the structural requirements for inhibition of AGE formation. Matsuda *et al.,* (2003) proposed that the number of hydroxyl groups at the 3′, 4′, 5 and 7 positions may play an important role in the potency of AGE formation inhibitor.

Table 3.4 IC_{50} Inhibitory activities values of prenylated flavonoids isolated from the root extract of *Sophora flavescens* against AGEs (Jung *et al.,* 2008b).

Flavonoid	AGEs	
	μgmL^{-1}	μM
Desmethylanhydroicartin (32)	104.3	294.6
8-Lavandulylkaempferol (33)	132.1	313.1
Kushenol C (34)	84.6	193.1
(2S)-3β,7,4´-Trihydroxy-5-methoxy-8-(γ,γ-dimethylallyl)-flavanone (35)	261.0	705.4
Aminoguanidin	115.7	1051.5

Several compounds including flavanonols, flavones, an aurone, a chalcone and simple phenolics have been isolated from the active ethyl acetate fraction of *Rhus verniciflua,* which showed concentration dependent inhibition against AGEs. The isolated compounds were identified as fustin (36), morin hydrate (37), fisetin (38), quercetin (39), sulfuretin (40), butein (41), ethyl gallate (42), and protocatechuic acid (43). The sulfuretin (40) and butein (41) showed the strongest AGEs inhibition, and the inhibitory potencies as expressed by IC_{50} values, were shown in table 5. It has been reported that the hydroxyl groups of flavones at the 3´-, 4´-, 5´-, and 7-positions increased the AGEs inhibitory activities and the methylation or glycosilation of the 3´- or 4´-hydroxyl group reduced the activity (Lee *et al.,* 2008).

Table 3.5 Inhibitory Effects of the Compounds Isolated from the Bark of *R.verniciflua* on AGEs (Lee *et al.* 2008).

Compounds	Conc. (μm)	%inhibition	$IC_{50}(\mu M)$
Aminoguanidine	2500	85.8±5.0	1450
	1250	49.1±1.7	
	625	11.8±4.2	
Fustin (36)	400	42.3±3.6	------
Morin Hydrate (37)	400	------	------
Fisetin (38),	400	-------	------
Quercetin (39)	400	23.6±2.4	-----
Sulfuretin (40)	400	79.9±0.3	124.0
	200	65.8±0.5	
	100	42.5±0.4	
Butein (41)	400	70.0±1.2	210.3
	200	47.8±1.4	
	100	27.6±1.3	
Protocatechuic Acid (43)	400	46.5±1.1	-----
Ethyl Gallate (42).	400	----	-----

It has been reported that the EtOAc extract of mustard leaf not only showed potent antiglycation activity and inhibitory effect on free radical-mediated protein damage *in vitro*, but also reduced the increased levels of superoxide and nitrite/nitrate, and protected against diabetic oxidative stress induced by streptozotocin *in vivo* (Yokozawa *et al.*, 2003). In addition, tomato paste strongly suppressed AGE formation chiefly due to one of its antioxidant components, rutin (Kiho *et al.*, 2004).

Lotus (*Nelumbo nucifera* Gaertn.) is an aquatic plant cultivated mostly in China and India but distributed throughout Asia. The young leaves, seeds and rhizome of the plant are used as vegetables while the matured leaves are used as functional foods. The inhibitory effect of lotus leaves, stamens, seeds, embryos and rhizomes on the formation of AGEs was investigated. Only the methanol extract of the leaves and stamens demonstrated good antiglycation activities with IC50 values of 110.5 µg/mL and 125.5 µg/mL respectively compared to the standard, aminoguanidine (Jung *et al.*, 2008a).

Musa paradisiaca belongs to the family musaceae. Commonly known as banana, methanolic extract and solvent fractions of banana were evaluated for their antiglycation activities using the BSA-glucose antiglycation model (Nisha *et al.*, 2014). Methanol extract as well as ethyl acetate, ether, water and butanol fractions displayed good antiglycation activities with IC_{50} 31, 118, 55 and 68 µg/mL respectively, and are Comparable to standard antiglycation agent aminoguanidine (IC_{50}: 61 µg/mL).

In another study Ramu *et al.,* 2014 reported that, Ethanolic extract of methanol-ethanol fraction of banana flower and two compounds (umbelliferone (1) and lupeol (2)) also inhibited the formation of glycation product. (umbelliferone (44) and lupeol (45)) can inhibit them in the range of 71–82%. It is worth mentioning that (umbelliferone (44) and lupeol (45)) exhibited higher inhibition compared to a known inhibitor aminoguanidine at diverse concentrations on 21-day incubation.

Two anthocyanins, cyanidin-3-α-*O*-rhamnoside(46), pelargonidin-3-α-*O*-rhamnoside(47), and quercitrin (quercetin-3-α-*O*-rhamnoside)(48), were isolated from methanolic extract of acerola (*Malpighia emarginata* DC) fruit. These polyphenols were evaluated for the AGE formation inhibitory activities. At the concentration of 0.3mg/mL all the three phenols shows the inhibitory activity, among the tested compounds quercetin-3-α-*O*-rhamnoside show better activity than amino guanidine (Hanamura *et al.,* 2005).

Anti-LDL glycative agents were investigated using aqueous extracts of *Psidium guajava* L. (PE), *Toona sinensis* Roem. (TE), *Momordica charantia* L. (ME) and *Graptopetalum paragugayene* E. Walther (GE). The inhibitory effect of PE on the AGEs formations induced by glucose at a concentration of 0.01 mg/mL was shown to reach 63.45%, comparing with

36.58% induced by glyoxal. Obviously, PE is able to impose a remarkable inhibitory effect on the AGEs formation. Taking AG as the positive control, the effectiveness as expressed in % inhibition on AGEs formation induced by glyoxal was found to be in the order: PE (36.58%)>TE (30.82%) >GE(19.28%)>ME (inactive) >AG (1.59%) (Hsieh *et al.*, 2005).

Bitter melon (*Momordica charantia* L.) is a plant which is consumed as food and used as ingredient in some Asian curries. A pilot study on the antiglycation potential of bitter melon was investigated in type 2 diabetic patients for 16 weeks (Trakoon-osot *et al.*, 2013). The study involved the consumption of 6.0 g dried fruit powder of bitter melon daily by the diabetic patients throughout the duration of the experiment, which resulted in significant reduction in the levels of glycated hemoglobin (HbA1c) and serum AGEs of the patients by 6.69% and 6.65% respectively.

The antiglycation property of polysaccharide fraction isolated from aqueous extract of fruit rind of pomegranate was investigated (Rout *et al,* 2007). The inhibition study for the production of AGEs was carried out in different concentrations (10 - 20 μg/mL) of polysaccharide fraction. It was able to inhibit the production AGEs by 28% in 10 μg/mL concentration as against the same concentrations of vitamin C, which resulted in 41% inhibition.

Aegle marmelos from the family of Rutaceae, also known as golden apple, bael apple, wood apple, and stone apple, is native to India. It is a commonly used food with varieties of biological properties. Methanolic extract of bael apple exhibited antiglycation property with an IC_{50} value of 60.14±1.43 μg/mL and that of standard compound ascorbic acid is 30.51±0.71 μg/mL (Prathapan *et al.*, 2012).

In a BSA-fructose antiglycation assay, aqueous extract of apple and green-tea fortified apple displayed anti-AGE formation activities of 15 and 48 mg/kg dry weight respectively (Lavelli *et al.*, 2011). Common juniper (*Juniperus communis* and *oblonga*) is an evergreen shrub which is endemic to Europe, Asia and North America. Asgary *et al.*, 2014 reported that, the inhibitory activity of the oils from fruits and branchlets of *Juniperus communis* subsp. *Hemisphaerica* against hemoglobin glycation. The highest inhibitory activity was observed with female branchlet oil (89.9%) followed by male branchlet (74.7%) and fruit (62.8%) oils. All tested oils showed ≥50% inhibitory activity against insulin glycation. The highest activity of male branchlet and female branchlet oils was observed at 600 μg/mL, concentration to 64.0% and 81.0% inhibition, respectively. In another study, Essential oils isolated from the fruits and branchlets of *Juniperus oblonga* inhibited the glycation of haemoglobin at all concentrations tested (200, 400 and 600 μg/mL) (Emami *et al.*, 2012).

Jariyapamornkoon *et al.*, 2013 reported that, the inhibition of AGEs by red grape (*Vitis vinifera* L.) skin extract. After 4 weeks of incubation, the grape extract (0.031-0.5 mg/mL) inhibited the formation of AGE by 55.23% to 63.52%. The extract (0.5 mg/mL) also reduced the level of fructosamine and carbonyl content generated by 10.5% and 41.7% respectively. Incubation with the 0.5 mg/mL extract also caused significant improvement (50.4%) in the level of protein thiol group and concomitant decrease (58.1%) in the carboxyl methylysine content.

Nine phenolic compounds have been isolated from the methanolic extract of ethyl acetate soluble fraction of *Cordia sinensis*, namely protocatechuic acid (43), *trans*-caffeic acid (49), methyl rosmarinate (50), rosmarinic acid (51), kaempferide-3-*O*-*β*-D-glucopyranoside (52), kaempferol-3-*O*-*β*-Dglucopyranoside (53), quercetin-3-*O*-*β*-D-glucopyranoside (54), kaempferide-3-*O*-α-Lrhamnopyranosyl (1→6)-*β*-D-glucopyranoside (55) and kaempferol-3-*O*-α-L-rhamnopyranosyl (1→6)-*β*-D-glucopyranoside (56). All the isolated compounds showed significant anti-glycation inhibitory activity and their % Inhibitory activities shown in table 6. Among them, methyl rosmarinate (50) shows better inhibitory activity (88.4%) than rutin (86%), this was used as standard (Al-Musayeib et al., 2011).

Table 3.6 % Inhibitory activities values of isolated from the methanolic extract of ethyl acetate soluble fraction of *Cordia sinensis* against AGEs (Al-Musayeib *et al.*, 2011).

Phenolic compounds	% Inhibition
Protocatechuic acid (43),	68.0
Trans-caffeic acid (49),	69.2
Methyl rosmarinate (50),	88.4
Rosmarinic acid (51),	87.3
Kaempferide-3-*O*-*β*-D-glucopyranoside (52),	76.5
Kaempferol-3-*O*-*β*-Dglucopyranoside (53),	74.0
Quercetin-3-*O*-*β*-D-glucopyranoside (54),	71.2
Kaempferide-3-*O*-α-Lrhamnopyranosyl(1→6)-*β*-D-glucopyranoside (55)	80.7
Kaempferol-3-*O*-α-L-rhamnopyranosyl(1→6)-*β*-D-glucopyranoside (56).	79.0
Rutin	86.0

Four flavonoid compounds (catechin (57), quercetin-3-*O*-galactoside(58), cyanidin-3-*O*-glucoside(59) and *para*-coumaric acid(60) were isolated from 80% ethanolic extract of berries *of Vaccinium vitis-idaea* L and assessed for their inhibitory effect on AGEs. Among, the tested compound quercetin-3-*O*-galactoside (58) shows the high inhibitory activity (6.16 ±1.15 µM) when compared with other. *para*-coumaric (60) acid does not show activities. (Beaulieu et al., 2010).

Psidium guajava L. is a tropical fruit and the leaves of which are used as a folk therapeutic in the treatment of diabetes and enteritis and its Potential of Ethyl Acetate fraction was demonstrated a potent antiglycative agent (Soman *et al.,* 2010). In another study, Guava leaf extract at the concentration of 50 μg/mL also exhibited strong inhibition (over 90%) of α-dicarbonyl compounds formation. Catechin (57), gallic acid (61), ferulic acid (62) and quercetin (39) (from the guava extract) also displayed over 80% inhibitory effect on α-dicarbonyl compounds formation while ferulic acid (62) did not. Both the extract and active compounds of guava leaf inhibited the formation of Amadori products (fructosamine) and AGEs from albumin in the presence of glucose. This α-dicarbonyl compounds formation was confirmed when the ethyl acetate extract of guava leaf exhibited IC_{50} value of 38.95 μg/mL for the inhibition of protein glycation, which is similar to the activity of standard antiglycation agent, aminoguanidine (IC_{50}: 33.82 μg/mL) (Wu *et al.,* 2009).

Administration of 100 and 200 mg/kg of Cornelian cherry extract to diabetic rats for 10 days significantly reduced the renal AGE level to 5.32 and 4.92 IU compared to 6.19 IU in diabetic control group (Yamabe *et al.,* 2007a). The renal AGE level of the diabetic rats administered 200 mg/kg cornelian cherry was similar to the group that received standard antiglycation agent, aminoguanidine. Administration of 20 mg/kg iridoid glycoside and low molecular weight polyphenol fractions of Cornelian cherry to streptozotocin-induced diabetic rats for 10 days, also showed that the iridoid glycosides fraction significantly reduced serum glycosylated protein (19.7 nmol/mg protein) and renal AGE (3.90 IU) compared to the diabetic control (21.5 nmol/mg protein and 4.45 IU respectively) while the polyphenol fractions caused down-regulation of receptor for advanced glycation end products (RAGE) to a value of 1.58 and 1.21-fold lower than the normal rats (Yamabe et al., 2007b).

Park *et al.,* 2012 reported that, the two iridoid glycoside morroniside (63) and loganin (64), and one polyphenol i.e., 7-*O*-galloyl-D-sedoheptulose (65) isolated from hot water extract of *Corni fructus. Corni fructus* extracts and tested for anti-glycation activity. Iridoid glycoside components, morroniside and loganin, showed low inhibitory activity than Trolox, known as an antioxidant. On the other hand, the inhibitory activity of 7-*O*-galloyl-D-sedoheptulose was higher (61.90% at 25μg/mL) than that of other references (Trolox and aminoguanidine).

Longan (*Dimocarpus longan* Lour.) is a tropical tree that produces exotic, attractive and edible fruits. Ultrasonic wave was used to extract the polysaccharides from longan fruit pericarp. The antiglycation activity of polysaccharides of longan fruit was investigated by using three ultrasonic factors: ultrasonic power (120–300 W), time (10–30min) and temperature (30–70^{0}C) (Yang *et al.,* 2009). The study showed that polysaccharides obtained after ultrasonic treatment under different conditions, exhibited potent antiglycation effect in BSA-glucose glycation system.

Morrone *et al.*, 2013 reported that the protective effect of hot water extract of passion fruit (*Passiflora manicata*) on protein glycation. To evaluate the effect of aqueous extract on protein glycation, an *in vitro* assay using a glycation-inducing reaction system with purified bovine albumin, fructose and glucose. Extract was added to this incubation system, the results show a significant inhibition of protein glycation at 1, 10 and 100 µg/mL concentrations.

Pomelo (*Citrus grandis* L.), which belongs to the family Rutaceae, is one of the most widely cultivated crops in Southeast Asia. The effect of aqueous methanol extract of shaddock fruit on the concentration of AGEs, fructosamine, carbonyl and carboxymethylysine was reported (Caengprasath *et al.*, 2013). Shaddock extract (0.25 – 2.00 mg/mL) significantly inhibited the formation of AGEs in concentration dependent manner to a maximum of 90.68% on the 28th day. The extract also reduced fructosamine concentration by 3.7, 9.9, 17.5 and 30% at 0.25, 0.50, 1.00 and 2.0 mg/mL respectively.

Rambutan (*Nephelium lappaceum* L.) is a tropical fruit which is native to South East Asia. Geraniin (66), an ellagitannin was identified as the major bioactive compound isolated from the ethanolic *Nephelium lappaceum* L. rind extract. Inhibition was investigated on AGEs using geraniin (66) (20 µg/mL) and *N. lappaceum* extract (40 µg/mL) while green tea extract (40 µg/mL) was used as the positive control. It was observed that both geraniin (66) and *N. lappaceum* ethanolic extract exhibited higher AGEs inhibition activity compared to the green tea throughout the 7-day incubation period (Palanisamy *et al.*, 2011).

Water apple (*Syzygium aqueum* Alston) is a tropical plant which originated from Malaysia and Indonesia. Manaharan *et al.*, 2012 reported that, the inhibitory effect of ethanolic leaf extract of water apple on the formation of AGEs. Inhibitory activity was shows at the incubation time of 7 days, 89% inhibition for ethanolic extract of *S. aqueum* leaf and 45% for green tea. Green tea was used as a positive control in this AGE inhibition assay.

Kokum (*Garcinia indica* Choicy) is an under exploited tree which is distributed throughout the tropical Asian and African countries. Garcinol (67), a poly isoprenylated benzophenone derivative, was isolated from ethanolic extract of *Garcinia indica* fruit rind. Garcinol suppressed the fluorescence formation at a concentration of 0.01 mM than quercetin, which was reported as a potent glycation inhibitor (Yamaguchi *et al.*, 2000).

Apples (*Malus domestica*) are one of the most important fruits in the world. In a BSA-fructose antiglycation assay, aqueous extract of apple band green-tea fortified apple displayed anti-AGE formation activities of 15 and 48 mg/kg dry weight respectively (Lavelli *et al.*, 2011).

Green tea extract could reduce age-related increase in collagen cross-linking and fluorescent products in C57BL/6 mice (Rutter *et al.*, 2003). and protect against protein oxidation and glycation mainly due to tannin components whose chemical structures were involved in the protective activity (Nakagawa et al., 2002) In addition, the inhibitory effect of green tea extract was compared with *Ilex paraguariensis* (IP) extract. Neither of them presented significant participation as inhibitors in the early phase of the glycation process based on the results from the SDS-PAGE. IP extract mainly inhibited the free-radical mediated conversion of Amadori products to AGEs with activity comparable to that of aminoguanidine, whereas green tea extract was weaker (Lunceford *et al.*, 2005).

Luobuma tea, prepared from the leaves of *Apocynum venetum* L., is a popular beverage in China. The aqueous extract from Luobuma tea was studied by the measurement of fluorescence AGEs formed in bovine serum saline with the addition of glucose. It showed obvious activity against AGE formation. Following further fractionations of the extract, seven polyphenolic compounds, i.e. (±)-gallocatechin (68), (-)-epigallocatechin (69), (±)-catechin (70), (-)-epicatechin (71), epicatechin-(4β-8)-gallocatechin (72), epigallocatechin-(4β-8)-epicatechin (73) and procyanidin B-2 (74) were isolated which presented more potent inhibitory effects against AGE formation than aminoguanidine. Their IC_{50} values are summarized in table 3.7. (Yokozawa *et al.*, 2004).

Table 3.7 IC_{50} (µM) values of isolated compounds from the leaves of *Apocynum venetum* L.against AGEs (Yokozawa *et al.*, 2004).

Isolated compounds	IC_{50} (µM)
(±)-Gallocatechin, (68),	19.8±0.8
(-)-Epigallocatechin (69),	9.1±0.2
(±)-Catechin, (70),	13.1±0.2
(-)-Epicatechin, (71),	17.4±0.2
Epicatechin-(4β-8)-gallocatechin (72),	14.9±0.2
Epigallocatechin-(4β-8)-epicatechin (73),	12.8±0.1
Procyanidin B-2 (74),	13.4±0.1
Amino guanidine	59.2±1.5

Lunceford *et al.*, 2005 reported the inhibition of AGE formation by the aqueous extract of yerba mate (*Ilex paraguariensis* St. Hil). Co-incubation of bovineserum albumin (BSA) and methylglyoxal with yerba mate extract caused a dose-dependent inhibition of glycation reaching up to 40% at 20 µL/mL of the extract, which implies good antiglycation effect.

The *in vitro* antiglycation and cross-link breaking potential of black tea from Sri Lanka was reported (Ratnasooriya *et al.*, 2014). Black tea brew exhibited high antiglycation (IC_{50}: 19.04 µg/mL) and AGEs cross-link breaking (IC_{50}: 82.89 µg/mL) activities, and these activities were similar to that of popular antiglycation agent, rutin.

Dendrobii (*Dendrobium huoshanense*) is another antiglycation tea plant which is endemic to Huoshan town, Anhui Province of China. It is used as spice in the preparation of foods such as soups and as herbal tea. The antiglycation activity of polysaccharides extracted from dendrobii has been reported (Li *et al.*, 2014). Polysaccharides from dendrobii inhibited the formation of amadori product in a dose-dependent manner to maximum of 72.54%, which was about 1.95 fold greater than that of aminoguanidine. The formation of intermediate dicarbonyl compound and AGEs was also decreased to a minimum of 51.9%, which is lower than that of aminoguanidine. The inhibition of glycation by these polysaccharides of dendrobii may be due to their antioxidant properties.

Screening was carried out by Hori *et al.*, 2012 on AGEs activity of 32 tea (*Camella sinensis*) samples and 81 herbal tea Samples. The IC_{50} of all 113 tea and herbal tea samples (1-hour and 3-minute extractions) against fluorescent AGEs formation in collagen were ranked. Samples with IC_{50} 20-fold less than that of aminoguanidine (IC_{50}= 0.40mg/mL) for both 3-minute and 1-hour extract were selected and classified under *Camellia sinensis* derived teas and non-*Camellia sinensis* derived teas (herbal teas) (IC_{50} values of shown in Figure 3.2).

The anti-glycation activity of four kinds of beans including mung bean, black bean, soybean and cowpea were evaluated. Aqueous alcohol extract of mung bean exhibited the strongest inhibitory activity against the formation of fluorescent advanced glycation end products (AGEs) in a bovine serum albumin (BSA)-glucose model, and the inhibitory activities of extracts of the four beans were found to be high. Subsequent HPLC analysis of mung bean extract revealed two major phenolics which were identified as vitexin (75) and isovitexin (76). In the anti-glycation assays, both vitexin (75) and isovitexin (76) showed significant inhibitory activities against the formation of AGEs induced by glucose or methylglyoxal with efficacies of over 85% at 100 µM (Penga *et al.*, 2008).

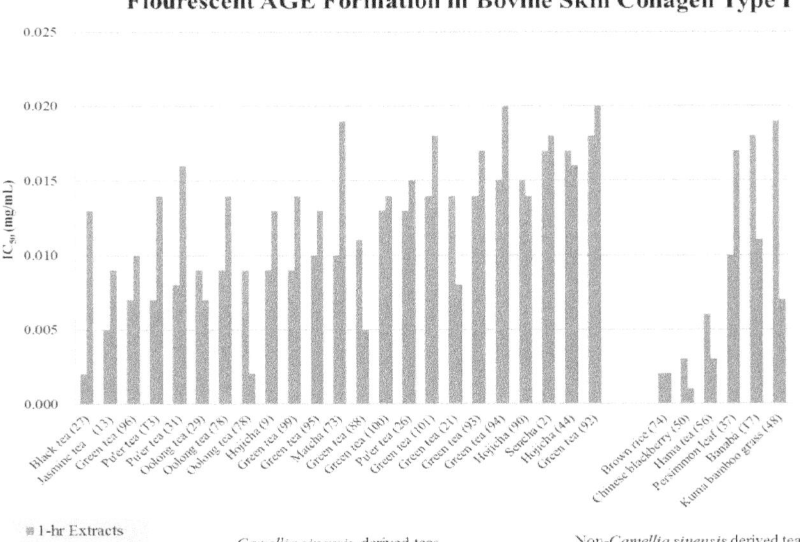

Figure 3.2 Inhibitory activity of selected teas and herbal teas (1-hour and 3-minute extracts) against fluorescent AGE formation in collagen. IC_{50} values are expressed in mg/ml. The samples are categorized as *Camellia sinensis*-derived teas or non-*Camellia sinensis*-derived teas (herbal teas). AGE; advanced glycation end product. IC_{50}: 50% inhibitory concentration (Hori *et al.*, 2012).

Cassiaside (77), rubrofusarin-6-O-β-D-gentiobioside (78) and toralactone-9-O-β-D-gentiobioside (79) belongs to naphthopyrone glucosides derivatives, isolated from butanol soluble extract of *Cassia tora* L. (sickle senna) seeds and isolated compound displayed antiglycation property when carried out the AGEs *in vitro assay*. Tested naphthopyrone glucosides derivatives showed better inhibition of AGE formation (IC_{50} value shown in table 8) than the standard antiglycation agent, aminoguanidine (Lee *et al.*, 2006). In another study, nine anthraquinones, aurantio-obtusin (80), chryso-obtusin (81), obtusin (82), chryso-obtusin-2-O-β -D-glucoside (83), physcion (84), emodin (85), chrysophanol (86), obtusifolin (87), and obtusifolin-2-O-β -D-glucoside (88), isolated from an EtOAc-soluble extract of the seeds of *Cassia tora* and evaluated their AR inhibiting activity. Among the tested, compounds 85 and 87 exhibited a significant inhibitory activity on AGEs formation with observed IC_{50} values of shown in table 9, in an AGEs-bovine serum albumin (BSA) assay by specific fluorescence. Further, compounds 85 and 87 inhibited AGEs-BSA formation more effectively than aminoguanidine, an AGEs inhibitor, by indirect AGEs-ELISA (Jang *et al.*, 2007).

Table 3.8 IC_{50} Inhibitory activities values of naphthopyrone glucosides derivatives isolated from the butanol seeds extract of *Cassia tora* against AGEs (Lee *et al.*, 2006).

Naphthopyrone glucosides	AGEs		
	Conc(µg/ml)	%inhibition	IC_{50} (µM)
Cassiaside (77)	10	25.4±0.7	
	25	40.9±3.8	32.2(76.7)
	50	70.6±1.5	
Rubrofusarin-6-*O*-β-D-gentiobioside (78)	10	38.5±1.5	
	25	54.3±2.5	20.3(34.1)
	50	85.9±1.4	
Toralactone-9-*O*-β-D-gentiobioside (79)	2.5	9.3±3.2	
	5	38.1±9.4	6.4(10.7)
	10	85.1±7.4	
Aminoguanidin	18.5	25.3±3.2	
	37	54.6±0.9	34.6(467)
	74	69.7±0.9	

Table 3.9 IC_{50} Inhibitory activities values of isolated compounds from the Compounds from the Seeds of *C. tora* against AGEs (Jang *et al.*, 2007).

Anthraquinones derivatives	IC_{50} (µM)
Aurantio-obtusin (80),	›1000
Chryso-obtusin-2-*O*-β -D-glucoside (83),	›1000
Emodin (85),	118
Obtusifolin (87),	28.9
Aminoguanidin	961

The *in vitro* antiglycation activity of common buckwheat hull (*Fagopyrum esculentum*) infusion was investigated (Zielinska *et al.*, 2013). The ready-to-drink buckwheat hull tea displayed lower inhibition (34.90%) of AGEs in BSA-glucose system compared to green tea. Lee *et al.* (2015) also reported the inhibitory effect of ethanol extract of tartary buckwheat (*Fagopyrum tataricum*) on the formation of AGEs, fructosamine (Amadori product) and dicarbonyl compounds. Ethanol extract (200 µg/mL) of tartary buckwheat exhibited strong inhibition of AGEs (83%), fructosamine (50%) and α-dicarbonyl compounds (65%) formation.

Turmeric extracts were evaluated for their ability to retard glycation reaction between albumin and glucose (Fig.3.1c). Turmeric extracts except hexane extract were potent to inhibit the glycation reaction. Similar to glucosidase inhibition, in antiglycation activity also ethyl acetate (IC50=0.09µg/mL) showed the highest potential followed by methanol (IC50=1.48µg/mL) and water (IC50=10.42µg/mL) extracts. Antiglycation potential of turmeric ethyl acetate extract was about 800 times higher than ascorbic acid (Lakshmi *et al.,* 2014).

The inhibition of protein glycation by ginger extract in an *in vitro* model was investigated (Rani *et al.,* 2011). Ethylacetate extract of ginger at varying concentrations (100-500 μg/mL) displayed dose-dependent inhibition of albumin glycation, which culminated in its IC_{50} value of 290.84 μg/mL for the antiglycation activity. In another study, Kazeem *et al.,* 2015 investigated the antiglycation effects of polyphenols extracted from ginger in streptozotocin-induced diabetic rats. Oral administration of 500 mg/kg of free and bound polyphenols of ginger to diabetic rats for 42 days significantly reduced the glycated haemoglobin (HbA1c) level (7.10%) compared to the diabetic control (10.33%). The formation of AGEs in the serum was also drastically decreased from 6.80 μg/mL in the diabetic control rats, to 1.98 μg/mL in the ginger-treated diabetic animals.

Kazeem et al., 2012, evaluate the antiglycation potential of 80% acetone extract of polyphenols spices; alligator pepper, ginger and nutmeg. All the extracts inhibited the glucose-mediated formation of fluorescent AGEs in a dose-dependent manner. At 1.0 mg/mL, all the extracts exhibited high inhibition towards the formation of AGEs which was retained by alligator pepper at all concentrations. Its inhibitory capacity was significantly different (P<0.05) compared to ginger and nutmeg at all concentrations tested. At 0.25 mg/mL, the antiglycation capacity of the extracts followed this order; alligator pepper (73.4%), nutmeg (55.5%), ginger (46.4%). alligator pepper had the lowest IC_{50} (0.125) compared to that of ginger (0.285) and curry (0.200).

The inhibition of AGEs formation by clove extract was investigated (Suantawee *et al.,* 2015). Clove extract (0.25 – 1.00 mg/mL) inhibited the formation of AGEs to a maximum of 95.2% as against the standard, aminoguanidine (91.5%). It also caused 72.8% reduction in the formation of N-carboxy methylysine (Suantawee *et al.,* 2015). Co-incubation of the clove extract with the glycation reaction mixture also decreased the formation of protein carbonyl content by 73.7%, as comparable to aminoguanidine (60.0%).

Leaf and inflorescence extracts from three *Ocimum* species and major metabolites there in including camphor(89), eucalyptol(90), α-pinene(91), β-ocimene(92), terpinolene(93), farnesene(94), β-caryophyllene(95), eugenol(96), and eugenol methyl ether (EME)(97) were evaluated for their *in vitro* anti-glycation activity using BSA-AGE fluorescence assay. Maximum inhibition of glycation was observed with *O. gratissimum* extract, which is rich of eugenol. Inflorescence and leaf extracts of *O. gratissimum* inhibited the formation of AGEs by 74% and 72%, respectively (Figure-3.3a). *O. tenuiflorum* leaf extracts rich in EME showed least (10%) inhibition of glycation (Figure-3.3a). *O. kilimandscharicum* and inflorescence extracts, rich in camphor and eucalyptol displayed significant inhibition of AGE formation, 46% and 42%, respectively (Figure-3.3a). Of all the metabolites assessed, eugenol displayed highest, 58% inhibition of glycation (Figure-3.3b). Other metabolites did not inhibit AGE formation significantly (Singh *et al.*, 2015).

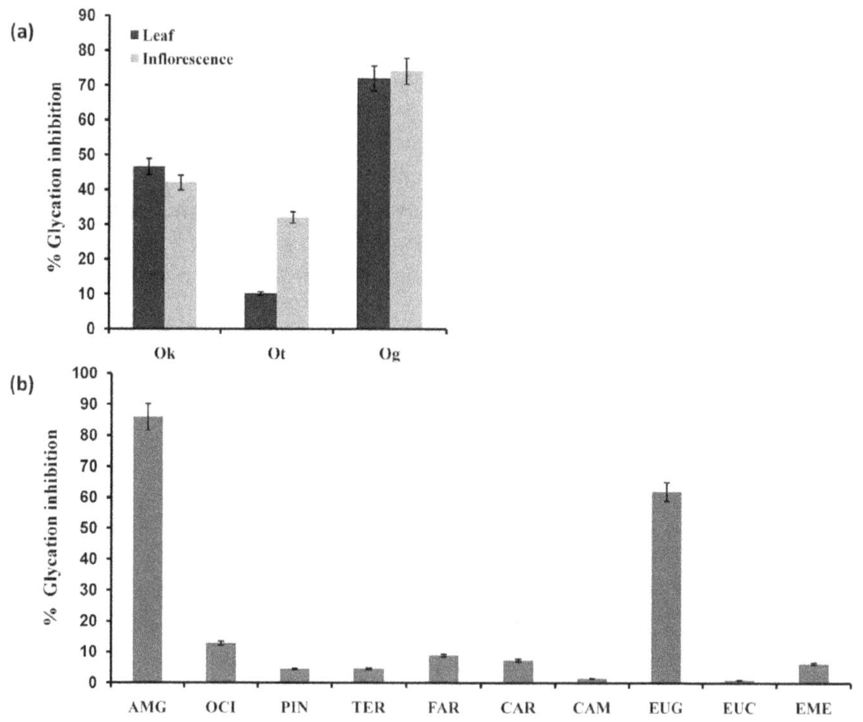

Figure 3.3 *In vitro* BSA-AGE inhibition assay. Glycation inhibition shown by (a) leaf and inflorescence extracts of *O. kilimandscharicum* (Ok), *O. tenuiflorum* (Ot), *O. gratissimum* (Og) and (b) standard compounds, aminoguanidine (AMG), ocimene (OCI), pinene (PIN), terpinolene (TER), farnesene (FAR), β – caryophyllene (CAR), camphor (CAM), eugenol (EUG), eucalyptol (EUC) and eugenol methyl ether (EME). (Singh *et al.*, 2015).

Methanolic extract of cumin seed was also tested for its inhibitory effect on glucose induced BSA glycation. Cumin extract exhibited concentration dependent inhibition of BSA glycation and subsequent formation of fluorescent glycation products, culminating in low IC_{50} of 1.17 mg/mL (Jagtap *et al.*, 2010).

An essential oil component cymene, extracted from several types of plants, has been routinely used as flavoring agent in the food industry. Fructosamine is a marker of early glycation. It can be seen that glycation of

BSA leads to large generation of fructosamine (almost 40-fold higher values). Cymene demonstrates a dose dependent decrease in the fructosamine level. The value of fructosamine by treating with cymene at 100 µM is comparable with a dose of 2 mM of aminoguanidine, implying that cymene is effective at a concentration that is twenty times less than aminoguanidine in preventing early glycation of proteins. (Joglekar *et al.,* 2014).

The antiglycation property of ethanolic extract of the leaves of black nightshade (*Solanum nigrum* L.), and two of its isolated compounds, solasonine (98) and solamargine (99) were investigated (Hou *et al.,* 2013). The result revealed that 95% ethanolic extract of black nightshade inhibited the generation of AGEs in a dose-dependent manner, via the lowering of fructosamine and α-dicarbonyl compounds formation (shown in Figure 3.4). Solasonine also exerted stronger antiglycation activity for attenuating AGEs, fructosamine and α-dicarbonyl compounds formation than solarmargine. This implies that black nightshade leaves possess antiglycation effects which may be due to the presence of solasonine.

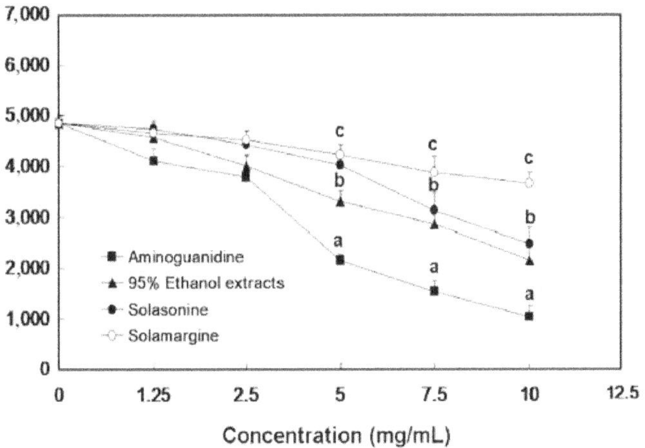

Figure 3.4 Anti-AGEs generations of 95% ethanolic extracts of black nightshade, solasonine, and solamargine. Data are indicated as mean±SD; Different superscripts are significantly different (p<0.05). (Hou, *et al.,* 2013).

Ho and Chang, 2012 reported that, the Inhibitory Effects of methanolic extracts of eight Spices on Advanced Glycation End products. In table 10, shows the Antiglycating capacities of spice extracts. The anti- glycating capacities of the spice extracts, given by IC_{50} declined in the order; cinnamon, thyme, turmeric, rosemary, basil, parsley, cumin and cardamom.

Table 3.10 IC_{50} (µM) values of the methanolic extract of Spices against AGEs (Ho and Chang, 2012).

Spices	(%) Inhibitory capacity200 (µg/mL).	IC_{50} (µM)
Cinnamon (1),	99.3±1.4	26.0
Thyme, (2),	94.9±0.3	44.2
Turmeric (3),	89.9±0.6	50.6
Rosemary (4),	91.1±1.9	58.8
Basil, (5),	80.7±0.9	83.7
Parsley (6),	74.5±1.5	99.1
Cumin (7),	81.6±0.9	111.6
Cardamom (8)	68.6±0.14	129.5
Amino guanidine(800µm)	102.9±2.2	--------

Nine compounds (protocatechuic acid (43), protocatechualdehyde (100), caffeic acid (101), ellagic acid (102), hispidin (103), davallialactone (104), hypolomin B (105), interfungin A (106), and inoscavin A (107)) isolated from the ethylacetate fraction of sangwhang *(Phellinus linteus)*, were evaluated for antiglycation activities and there IC_{50} values shown in table 11 (Lee *et al.*, 2008). Davallialactone (50.2%), interfungin A (63.1%), and inoscavin A (45.7%) exhibited inhibitory effect on HbA1c formation, while protocatechualdehyde (IC_{50}: 144.28 µM), davallialactone (IC_{50}: 158.66 µM) and inoscavin A (IC_{50}: 213.15 µM) prevented methylglyoxal-mediated protein modification. However, only interfungin A (IC_{50}: 1.15 mM) inhibited protein cross-links formation even better than aminoguanidine (IC_{50}: 11.93 mM). Therefore, Sangwhang displayed good inhibitory potential against AGEs formation which is due mainly to the presence of interfungin A.

Table 3.11 IC_{50} (µM) values of isolated from the methanolic extract of ethyl acetate soluble fraction of *Phellinus linteus* against AGEs (Lee *et al.*, 2008).

Isolated compounds	IC_{50} (µM)
Protocatechuic acid (43),	-----
Protocatechualdehyde (100),	144.28
Caffeic acid (101),	›1089.33
Ellagic acid (102),	334.74
Hispidin (103),	------
Davallialactone (104),	158.66
Hypholomine B (105),	428.00
Interfungins A (106)	213.15
Inoscavin A (107).	261.30
Amino guanidine	921.94

The methanolic extracts of Finger millet (*Eleusine coracana*) and Kodo millet (*Paspalum scrobiculatum*) were found to be useful for protection from glycation and cross-linking of collagen (Hegde *et al.,* 2002).

Among extracts of 34 spices, the methanol extract of thyme (*Thymus vulgaris*) showed the strongest activity in the inhibition of glycation of bovine serum albumin (BSA). Four flavonoids (quercetin (39), eriodictyol (108), 5,6,4-*O*-trihydroxy-7,8,3-*O*-trimethoxyflavone (109) and cirsilineol (110)) were isolated from thyme. Inhibitory activities of four flavonoids were evaluated on the formation of AGEs. In the fluorimetry method, quercetin (39), and eriodictyol (108) prevented the formation of AGEs just like aminoguanidine, a known authentic inhibitor (Morimitsu *et al.,* 1995).

Eight flavonoids and two novel indole alkaloids isolated from water soluble fraction of water-soluble fraction of matured seed skins of peanuts, *Arachis hypogaea* L. Two new flavonoid glycosides have been identified as isorhamnetin   3-O-[2-O-β-glucopyranosyl-6-O-α-rhamnopyranosyl]-β-glucopyranoside (112) and 3′, 5, 7-trihydroxyisoflavone-4′-methoxy-3′-O-β-glucopyranoside (114). These isolated flavonoids were evaluated for their protein glycation inhibitory effects. The AGEs inhibitory effects of tested compounds IC_{50} values were shown in Table 3.12 (Lou *et al.,* 2001).

Table 3.12 % Inhibitory activities values of isolated compounds from peanut skins against AGEs (Lou *et al.,* 2001).

Isolated compounds	% Inhibition
Quercetin-3-*O*-[2-*O*-β-xylopyranosyl-6-O-α-rhamnopyranosyl]-β-glucopyranoside (111)	46.64 ± 7.98
Isorhamnetin 3-*O*-[2-*O*-β-glucopyranosyl-6-O-α-rhamnopyranosyl]-β-glucopyranoside (112)	103.87 ± 12.76
Isorhamnetin 3-*O*-[2-*O*-β-xylopyranosyl-6-O-α-rhamnopyrano-syl]-β-glucopyranoside (113)	98.41 ± 11.66
3′, 5, 7-trihydroxyisoflavone-4′-methoxy-3′-O-β-glucopyranoside (114)	181.20 ± 18.62
3,5,7-trihydroxy-4-methoxyisoflavone (115)	185.23 ± 13.64
Rutin (116)	21.85 ± 4.12
Isorhamnetin-3-*O*-rutinoside (117)	35.20 ± 3.23
Quercetin-3-O-β-glucopyranoside (118)	35.20 ± 3.23
AG	1.4mM

From the brown alga, *Eisenia bicyclis*, a new phloroglucinol derivative 1-(3′,5′-dihydroxyphenoxy)-7-(2″,4″,6″-trihydroxyphenoxy)-2,4,9-trihydroxydibenzo-1,4dioxin (119), and two known compounds eckol (120) and dieckol (121) were isolated and the inhibitory effects of the isolated compounds on glycation were tested by ELISA. Inhibition was found to be

91.1% for a new phloroglucinol derivative, 96.2% for eckol, 86.7% for dieckol, and 76.0% for aminoguanidine at 1 mM (Okada *et al.*, 2004).

Origanum majorana L. (majorana) is an herbaceous and perennial plant native to southern Europe and the Mediterranean. For food uses, majorana is employed to flavor sausages, meats, salads, soups and spice in many countries. Gutierrez 2012 determine the inhibitory effect of the methanol extract of *O. majorana* on AGEs formation. *O. majorana* extract, and aminoguanidine exhibited higher inhibitory activity against AGEs formation after incubation at 37°C for 15 days, with an IC_{50} value of 0.310, and 0.323 mg/mL, respectively.

To confirm the potent inhibitory effects of aqueous extract of Chrysanthemum species (*C. morifolium* R. and *C. indicum* L.) on suppress AGE formation in BSA/glucose and BSA/fructose systems. Both Chrysanthemum species inhibited the formation of total AGEs after one week of incubation in BSA/glucose and BSA/fructose systems. The inhibitory effects of Chrysanthemum species at concentrations of 5.0 mg/mL were stronger than amino guanidine at concentrations of 1 mM as a positive control (Tsuji-Naito *et al.*, 2009).

The inhibitory effect of eleven 60% ethanolic herbal extracts on AGEs formation was carried out. The results of AGEs formation inhibition were summarized in table 13 indicated that the inhibitory strengths of herbal extracts were different from each other. It showed that the AGEs formation inhibitory activity of *Flos Sophorae Immaturus*, *Radix Scutellariae* and *Rhizoma Anemarrhenae* were better than others in the BSA/glucose (fructose) system by fluorescene analysis. (Hou *et al.*, 2014).

Table 3.13 The AGEs formation inhibition capacities of eleven kinds of herbal extracts. (Hou *et al.*, 2014).

Extracts	% inhibition
Amino guanidine	88.26±0.84
Flos Sophorae Immaturus	101.59±0.1
Radix Scutellariae	97.43±3.42
Cortex Cinnamomi	66.18±0.66
Folium Acanthopanacis Senticosi	51.33±0.38
Fructus Corni	53.94±0.82
Fructus Schisandrae Chinensis	61.11±1.30
Radix Glycyrrhizae	25.41±3.83
Rhizoma Anemarrhena	89.62±2.57
Radix Rehmanniae Praeparata	45.76±0.50
Radix Salviae Miltiorrhizae	36.01±0.52
Radix Paeoniae Rubra	70.92±0.87

Grzegorczyk-Karolak *et al.,* 2016 reported that, the ability of *Scutellaria altissima* and *S. alpina* extracts to inhibit AGE formation was evaluated by using the antiglycation assay, in which bovine serum albumin served as the model protein and glucose and fructose as the glycating agents. In general, *S. alpina* extracts showed a higher inhibitory effect than the extracts of *S. altissima.* Both *S. alpina* extracts presented more than 70% inhibition of AGE formation at a concentration of 100 µg/mL. From the extract identified the main metabolites i.e., flavonoids (baicalin (122), wogonoside (123), luteolin (124), luteolin-7-O-β-D-glucoside (125)) and one phenylethanoid (verbascoside) and carried out the their antiglycation capacity. Baicalin exhibited the highest antiglycation activity, followed by luteolin.

Harris *et al.,* 2011 reported that, the 80% ethanolic extracts of 17 medicinal plants were assessed for inhibitory effects on *in vitro* AGE formation through fluorometric and immune chemical detection of fluorescent AGEs and N^{ε}-(carboxymethyl)lysine adducts of albumin (CML-BSA), respectively. Most extracts inhibited fluorescent AGE formation with IC_{50} values ranging from 0.4-38.6 µg/mL and all the extracts reduce CML-BSA formation but to differing degrees. The antiglycation activities of Cree medicinal plant extracts and their reduced CML-BSA formation are summarized in table 3.14.

Table 3.14 Summary of the antiglycation activities of Cree medicinal plant extracts. (Harris *et al.,* 2011).

S.No.	Species (Family)	Part used	Family	IC_{50} (µg/mL) AGEs	Inhibition CML
1.	*Abies balsamea* (L.) Mill.		Pinaceae	34.2±12.5	38.3±8.0
2.	*Alnus incana subsp.* rugosa (Du Roi) R. T.Clausen		Betulaceae	N/A	72.3±6.4
3.	*Gaultheria hispidula* (L.) Muhl.		Ericaceae	1.5±0.2	67.8±5.7
4.	*Juniperus communis* L.		Cupressaceae	5.4±1.6	61.7±4.7
5.	*Kalmia angustifolia* L.		Ericaceae	1.5±0.5	72.3±4.6
6.	*Larix laricina* Du Roi (K. Koch)		Pinaceae	N/A	48.3±5.4
7.	*Lycopodium clavatum* L.		Lycopodiaeae	I/A	20.2±7.5
8.	*Picea glauca* (Moench.) Voss		Pinaceae	6.2±0.6	65.9±5.0
9.	*Picea mariana* (P. Mill) BSP		Pinaceae	2.1±0.2	64.5±7.9
10.	*Pinus banksiana* Lamb.		Pinaceae	1.5±0.2	76.2±7.8
11.	*Populus balsamifera* L.		Salicaceae	21.9±9.7	48.0±11.4

Table 3.14 *Contd...*

S.No.	Species (Family)	Part used	Family	IC$_{50}$ (µg/mL) AGEs	Inhibition CML
12.	*Rhododendron groenlandicum* (Oeder) Kron & Judd		Ericaceae	7.0±1.7	55.7±5.3
13.	*Rhododendron tomentosum* ssp. Subarcticum (Harjama) G. Wallace		Ericaceae	1.2±0.4	82.0±2.3
14.	*Salix planifolia* Pursh		Salicaceae	0.4±0.2	86.9±1.5
15.	*Salix planifolia* Pursh		Sarraceniaceae	38.6±1.9	67.8±1.7
16.	*Sorbus decora* (Sarg.) C. K. Schneid		Rosaceae	I/A	63.5±1.8
17.	*Vaccinium vitis-idaea* L.		Ericaceae	10.8±2.1	32.8±5.2
	Quercetin			1.8±0.7	85.8±3.7

Nawarathne Kalka (NK) is a similar poly herbal formulation which is used in Traditional Sri Lankan System of Medicine. This particular preparation contains components originating from 14 different plant species with honey and it is mainly prescribed for gastrointestinal tract disorders such as diarrhea, abdominal pain, haematochezia, indigestion as well as for rheumatoid arthritis (RA) and other inflammatory conditions. The ingredients and proportions of each component in NK and the parts of the plants used for its preparation are stated in Table 3.15. The aqueous extract of NK showed effective inhibitory action on the formation of AGEs with The EC$_{50}$ values obtained for the dose response curves corresponding to Week 1, 2 and Week 3 were 116±19 µg/mL, 125±35 µg/mL and 84 ±28 µg/mL respectively (Fernando *et al.*, 2016).

Table 3.15 Ingredients and proportions of Nawarathne Kalka (Fernando *et al.*, 2016).

Ingredients of Nawarathne Kalka	Part of the plant	Proportions (weightbasis)
Cedrus deodara (Vernacularname (VN): Devadara)	Bark	1
Cuminum cyminum (VN:Suduru)	seeds	1
Eugenia caryophylla (VN:Karabu)	Flower buds	1
Ferula asafetida (VN: Perunkayam)	resin	1
Glycyrrhiza glabra (VN: Valmi)	Stem	1
Myristica fragrans (VN: Sadikka)	Dried kernel of the seed	1
Nigella sativa (VN: Kaluduru)	Seeds	1
Picrorhiza kurroa (VN: Katukarosana)	Roots	1
Piper longum (VN: Thippili)	Dried fruit	1
Trachyspermum roxburghianum(VN:Asamodagum)	Seeds	1

Table 3.15 *Contd...*

Ingredients of Nawarathne Kalka	Part of the plant	Proportions (weightbasis)
Vernonia anthelmintica(VN: Sanninayam)	Seeds	1
Zingiber officinale (VN:Inguru)	Rhizome	1
Terminalia bellirica (VN: Bulu)	Fruit (outercover)	13
Terminalia chebula (VN: Aralu)	Fruit (outercover)	26
Honey	------	50

References

Ahmad MS, N Ahmed. J. Antiglycation properties of aged garlic extract: possible role in prevention of diabetic complications j. Nutr. 2006; 136: 796–799.

Ahmed N. 2005. Advanced glycation end products - Role in pathology of diabetic complications. *Diabetes Research and Clinical Practice* 67: 3-21.

Al-Musayeib N, Shagufta Perveen, Itrat Fatima, Muhammad Nasir and Ajaz Hussain. Antioxidant, Anti-Glycation and Anti-Inflammatory Activities of Phenolic Constituents from *Cordia sinensis. Molecules* 2011, *16*, 10214-10226.

Asgary S, GA Naderi1, MR Shams Ardekani, A Sahebkar, A Airin, S Aslani,T. Kasher, SA Emami. Inhibition of protein glycation by essential oils of branchlets and fruits of *Juniperus communis* subsp. *Hemisphaerica*. Research in Pharmaceutical Sciences, 2014; 9(3): 179-185.

Beaulieu LP, Cory S. Harris, Ammar Saleem, Alain Cuerrier, Pierre S. Haddad, Louis C. Martineau, Steffany A.L. Bennett, John T. Arnason. Inhibitory Effect of the Cree Traditional Medicine Wiishichimanaanh (*Vaccinium vitis-idaea*) on Advanced Glycation Endproduct Formation: Identifi cation of Active Principles. Phytother. Res. 2010; 24: 741–747.

Caengprasath N, Ngamukote S, Makynen K, Adisakwattana S. The protective effects of pomelo extract (*Citrus grandis* l. Osbeck) against fructose-mediated protein oxidation and glycation. *EXCLI Journal* 2013; 12: 491-502.

Daroux M, Prevost G, Maillard-Lefebvre H, Gaxatte C, D'agati VD, Schmidt AM, Boulanger, E. 2010. Advanced glycation end-products: Implications for diabetic and non-diabetic nephropathies. *Diabetes and Metabolism* 36: 1-10.

Emami SA, Sedigheh Asgary, Gholam A. Naderi,Mohammad R. S. Ardekani, Sanaz Aslani, Atousa Airin,Taghi Kasher, Amirhossein Sahebkar. Investigation of antioxidant and anti-glycation properties of essential oils from fruits and branchlets of *Juniperus oblonga*. Brazilian Journal of Pharmacognosy. 2012; 22(5): 985-993.

Fernando CD, Diyathi TK, Sachith DG, Dilusha MC, Prabuddhi K, Chandani U, Pathirage KP. Inhibitory action on the production of advanced glycation end products (AGEs) and suppression of free radicals in vitro by a Sri Lankan polyherbal formulation Nawarathne Kalka. BMC Complementary and Alternative Medicine 2016; 16:197-104.

Grzegorczyk-Karolak Izabela, Krzysztof Goła̗b, Jakub Gburek, Halina Wysokin´ ska and Adam Matkowski. Inhibition of Advanced Glycation End-Product Formation and Antioxidant Activity by Extracts and Polyphenols from Scutellaria alpina L. and S. altissima L. Molecules 2016, 21, 739-749.

Gugliucci A, T Menini. The botanical extracts of Achyrocline satureoides and *Ilex paraguariensis* prevent methylglyoxal-induced inhibition of plasminogen and antithrombin III. Life Sciences. 2002; 72*(3):* 279-292.

Gutierrez RMP. Inhibition of Advanced Glycation End-Product Formation by Origanum majorana L. *In Vitro* and in Streptozotocin-Induced Diabetic Rats. Evidence-Based   Complementary   and   Alternative   Medicine. 2012;doi:10.1155/2012/598638.

Hanamura T, Hagiwara T, Kawagishi H. Structural and functional characterization of polyphenols isolated from acerola (Malpighia emarginata DC.) fruit. Biosci Biotechnol Biochem. 2005; 69(2): 280-286.

Harris CS, Louis-Philippe Beaulieu, Marie-Hélène Fraser, Kristina L. McIntyre, Patrick L. Owen,Louis C. Martineau, Alain Cuerrier, Timothy Johns, Pierre S. Haddad, Steffany A.L. Bennett,John T. Arnason.Inhibition of Advanced Glycation End Product Formation by Medicinal Plant Extracts Correlates with Phenolic Metabolites and Antioxidant Activity. Planta Med 2011; 77: 196–204.

Hegde P, Chandrakasan G, Chandra T. Inhibition of collagen glycation and crosslinking in vitro by methanolic extracts of Finger millet (*Eleusine coracana*) and Kodo millet (*Paspalum scrobiculatum*). J Nutr Biochem. 2002; 13(9): 517-521.

Ho SC, Pei-Wen Chang. Inhibitory Effects of Several Spices on Inflammation Caused by Advanced Glycation Endproducts. American Journal of Plant Sciences. 2012; 3: 995-1002.

Hori M, Yagi M, Keitaro N, Akihiko S, Mari O, Yoshikazu Y. Inhibition of Advanced Glycation End Product Formation by Herbal Teas and Its Relation to Anti-Skin Aging. Anti-Aging Medicine 2012; 9 (6) : 135-148.

Hou GY, Lu Wang, Shu Liu, Feng-Rui Song, Zhi-Qiang Liu. Inhibitory effect of eleven herbal extracts on advanced glycation end products formation and aldose reductase activity. Chinese Chemical Letters 2014; 25, 1039-1043.

Hou TH, Jen-Ping Chung, Shang-Shan Chen, and Tsu-Liang Chang. Antioxidation and Antiglycation of 95% Ethanolic Extracts Preparedfrom the Leaves of Black Nightshade (Solanum nigrum). Food Sci. Biotechnol. 2013; 22(3): 839-844.

Hsieh CL, Yuh-Charn Lin, Wang-Sheng Ko, Chiung-Hui Peng, Chien-Ning Huange, Robert Y. Peng. Inhibitory effect of some selected nutraceutic herbs on LDL glycation induced by glucose and glyoxal. Journal of Ethnopharmacology. 2005; 10: 2357–363.

Hsieh CL, Yuh-Charn Lin, Wang-Sheng Ko, Chiung-Hui Peng,ChienNing Huang, Robert Y. Peng. Inhibitory effect of some selected nutraceutic herbs on LDL glycation induced by glucose and glyoxal. Journal of Ethnopharmacology 2005; 102: 357-363.

Imai J, Ide N, S. Nagae, T. Moriguchi, H. Matsuura, Y. Itakura. Antioxidant and Radical Scavenging Effects of Aged Garlic Extract and its Constituents. Planta Med. 1994; 60(5): 417-420.

Jagtap AG, PB Patil. Antihyperglycemic activity and inhibition of advanced glycation end product formation by Cuminum cyminum in streptozotocin induced diabetic rats. Food and Chemical Toxicology. 2010; 48: 2030–2036.

Jalaluddin Mohd Ashraf, Saheem Ahmad,Inho Choi, Nashrah Ahmad, Mohd Farhan, Godovikova Tatyana, Uzma Shahab. Recent Advances in Detection of AGEs:Immunochemical, Bioanalytical and Biochemical Approaches. International Union of Biochemistry and Molecular Biology 2015; 67(12): 897–913.

Jang DS, Ga Young Lee, Young Sook Kim, Yun Mi Lee, Chan-Sik Kim, Jeong Lim Yoo, Jin Sook Kim. Anthraquinones from the Seeds of *Cassia tora* with Inhibitory Activity on Protein Glycation and Aldose Reductase. *Biol. Pharm. Bull.* 2007; 30(11): 2207—2210.Es

Jang DS, Jong Min Kim,Yun Mi Lee, Young Sook Kim, Joo-Hwan Kim, and Jin Sook Kim. Puerariafuran, a New Inhibitor of Advanced Glycation End Products (AGEs) Isolated from the Roots of *Pueraria lobata*. Chem. Pharm. Bull. 2006; 54(9): 1315—1317.

Jariyapamornkoon N, Sirintorn Yibchok-anun, Sirichai Adisakwattana. Inhibition of advanced glycation end products byred grape skin extract and its antioxidant activity. Complementary and Alternative Medicine. 2013; 13:171-179.

Joglekar MM, Shrimant N Panaskar, Akalpita U Arvindekar. Inhibition of advanced glycation end product formation by cymene – A common food constituent. Journal of Functional Foods. 2014; 6: 107-115.

Jung HA, Jung YJ, Yoon NY *et al.* 2008a. Inhibitory effect of *Nelumbo nucifera* leaves on rat lens aldose reductase, advanced glycation endproducts formation and oxidative stress. *Food Chem Toxicol* 46: 3818-3826.

Jung HA, Yoon NY, Kang SS *et al.* 2008b. Inhibitory activities of prenylated flavonoids from *Sophora flavescens* against aldose reductase and generation of advanced glycation endproducts. *J Pharm Pharmacol* 60: 1227-1236.

Kang KS, Hyun Young Kim, Noriko Yamabe, Ryoji Nagai, Takako Yokozawa. Protective effect of *Sun Ginseng* against Diabetic Renal Damage. *Biol. Pharm. Bull.* 2006; 29(8): 1678-1684.

Kazeem MI, Akanji MA, Hafizur Rahman M, Choudhary MI. Antiglycation, antioxidant and toxicological potential of polyphenol extracts of alligator pepper, ginger and nutmeg from Nigeria. Asian Pacific Journal of Tropical Biomedicine 2012; 727-732.

Kazeem MI, Akanji MA, Yakubu MT, Ashafa AOT. Antiglycation and hypolipidemic effects of polyphenols from *Zingiber officinale* Roscoe (Zingiberaceae) in streptozotocin-induced diabetic rats. *Tropical Journal of Pharmaceutical Research*. 2015; 14: 55-61.

Kiho T, Usui S, Hirano K, Aizawa K, Inakuma T. Tomato paste fraction inhibiting the formation of advanced glycation end-products. Biosci., Biotechnol., Biochem., 2004; 68: 200–205.

Kim HY, Byung Ho Moon, Hak Ju Lee, Don Ha Choi. Flavonol glycosides from the leaves of *Eucommia ulmoides* O. with glycation inhibitory activity. Journal of Ethnopharmacology. 2004; 93: 227–230.

Kim HY, K Kim. Protein Glycation Inhibitory and Antioxidative Activities of Some Plant Extracts in Vitro. J. Agric. Food Chem. 2003; 51: 1586–1591.

Kim J, Chan-Sik Kim, Young Sook Kim, IK Soo Lee, Jin Sook Kim. Jakyakgamcho-Tang and Its Major Component, Paeonia Lactiflora, Exhibit Potent Anti-Glycation Properties. J Exerc Nutrition Biochem. 2016; 20 (4): 60-64.

Kim JM, Yun Mi Lee, Ga Young Lee, Dae Sik Jang, Ki Hwan Bae, and Jin Sook Kim. Constituents of the Roots of *Pueraria Lobata* Inhibit Formation of Advanced Glycation End Products (AGEs). Arch Pharm Res. 2006; 29(10): 821-825.

Lavelli V, Corey M, Kerr W, Vantaggi C. Stability and anti-glycation properties of intermediate moisture apple products fortified with green tea. *Food Chemistry* 2011; 127: 589-595.

Lavelli V, Mark Corey, William Kerr, Claudia Vantaggi. Stability and anti-glycation properties of intermediate moisture apple products fortified with green tea. Food Chemistry. 2011; 127: 589–595.

Lee CC, Lee BH, Lai YJ. Antioxidation and antiglycation of *Fagopyrum tataricum* ethanol extract. Journal of Food Science and Technology. 2015; 52: 1110-1116.

Lee EH, Song DG, Lee JY *et al.* 2008. Inhibitory effect of the compounds isolated from *Rhus verniciflua* on aldose reductase and advanced glycation endproducts. *Biol Pharma Bull* 31(8): 1626-1630.

Lee GY, Dae Sik Jang, Yun Mi Lee, Jong Min Kim, Jin Sook Kim. Naphthopyrone glucosides from the seeds of*Cassia tora* with inhibitory activity on advanced glycation end products (AGEs) formation. Archives of Pharmacal Research. 2006; 29: 587-590.

Lee YS, Young-Hee Kang, Ju-Young Jung, Sanghyun Lee, Kazuo Ohuchi, Kuk Hyun SHIN, Il-Jun Kang, Jung Han Yoon Park, Hyun-Kyung Shin, Soon Sung Lim. Protein Glycation Inhibitors from the Fruiting Body of *Phellinus linteus*. Biol. Pharm. Bull. 2008; 31(10): 1968-1972.

Lekshmi PC, Ranjith A, Nisha VM, A Nirmala Menon, KG Raghu. *In vitro* antidiabetic and inhibitory potential of turmeric (*Curcuma longa* L) rhizome against cellular and LDL oxidation and angiotensin converting enzyme. J Food Sci Technol. 2014; 51: 3910-3917.

Li XL, Xiao JJ, Zha XQ, Pan LH, Asghar MN, Luo JP. Structural identification and sulphated modification of anantiglycation *Dendrobium huoshanense* polysaccharide. *Carbohydrate Polymers* 2014; 106: 247-254.

Lou H, Huiqing Yuan, Yoshimitsu Yamazaki, Tsutomu Sasaki, Syuichi Oka. Alkaloids and Flavonoids from Peanut Skins. Planta Med. 2001: 67; 345-349.

Lunceford N, Alejandro Gugliucci. Ilex paraguariensis extracts inhibit AGE formation more efficiently than green tea. Fitoterapia. 2005: 76; 419– 427.

Lunceford N, Gugliucci A. *Ilex paraguariensis* extracts inhibit AGE formation more efficiently than green tea. Fitoterapia, 2005; 76: 419–427.

Manaharan T, Appleton D, Cheng HM, Palanisamy UD. Flavonoids isolated from *Syzygium aqueum* leaf extract as potential antihyperglycaemic agents. *Food Chemistry* 2012; 132: 1802-1807.

Matsuda H, Wang T, Managi H, Yoshikawa M. Structural requirements of flavonoids for inhibition of protein glycation and radical scavenging activities. *Bioorg. Med. Chem.* 2003; 11: 5317–5323.

Monnier VM, Mustata GT, biemel KL, Rheil O, Lederer MO, Zhenyu D, Sell DR. Cross-linking of the extracellular matrix by the Maillard reaction in aging and diabetes: An update on "a puzzle nearing resolution". *Annals of New York Academy of Science* 2005; 1043: 533-534.

Morimitsu Y, Kazunari Yoshida, Sachiko Esaki, Akira Hirota. Protein Glycation Inhibitors from Thyme (Thymus vulgaris). Biosci. Biotech. Biochem. 1995; 59 (11): 2018-2021.

Morrone MS, Adriano Martimbianco de Assisa, Ricardo Fagundes da Rocha, Juciano Gasparotto, Andressa Córneo Gazola, Geison Modesti Costa, Silvana Maria Zucolotto,Leonardo H. Castellanos, Freddy A. Ramos, Eloir Paulo Schenkel, Flávio Henrique Reginatto, Daniel Pens Gelain, José C.F. Moreira. Passiflora manicata (Juss.) aqueous leaf extract protects against reactive oxygen species and protein glycation in vitro and ex vivo models. Food and Chemical Toxicology. 2013; 60: 45–51.

Nakagawa T, Takako Yokozawa, Young Ae Kim and Ki Sung K. Activity of Wen-Pi-Tang, and Purified Constituents of Rhei Rhizoma and Glycyrrhizae Radix againstGlucose-Mediated Protein Damage. The American Journal of Chinese Medicine. 2005; 33: 817–829.

Nakagawa T, Yokozawa T, Terasawa K, Shu S, Juneja LR. Protective Activity of Green Tea against Free Radical- and Glucose-Mediated Protein Damage. Agric. Food Chem., 2002; 50: 2418–2422.

Nisha P, S. Mini. *In vitro* antioxidant and antiglycation properties of methanol extract and its different solvent fractions of *musa paradisiaca* l. (cv. Nendran) inflorescence. international journal of food properties. 2014; 17: 399–409.

Okada Y, Akiko Ishimaru, Ryuichiro Suzuki, and Toru Okuyama.A New Phloroglucinol Derivative from the Brown Alga *Eisenia bicyclis*: Potential for the Effective Treatment of Diabetic Complications. J. Nat. Prod. 2004; 67: 103-105.

Palanisamy UD, Lai Teng Ling, Thamilvaani Manaharan, David Appleton. Rapid isolation of geraniin from Nephelium lappaceum rind waste and its anti-hyperglycemic activity. Food Chemistry. 2011; 127: 21–27.

Park CH, Takashi Tanaka, Hyun Young Kim, Jong Cheol Park, and Takako Yokozawa. Protective Effects of Corni Fructus against Advanced Glycation Endproducts and Radical Scavenging. Evidence-Based Complementary and Alternative Medicine. 2012; doi:10.1155/2012/418953.

Penga X, Zongping Zhenga, Ka-Wing Chenga, Fang Shan, Gui-Xing Ren, Feng Chen, Mingfu Wang. Inhibitory effect of mung bean extract and its constituents isovitexin on the formation of advanced glycation endproducts. Food Chemistry. 2008; 106: 475–481.

Prathapan A, Mahesh S. Krishna, V.M. Nisha, A. Sundaresan, K.G. Raghu. Polyphenol rich fruit pulp of *Aegle marmelos* (L.) Correa exhibits nutraceutical properties to down regulate diabetic complications-An in vitro study. Food Research International. 2012; 48: 690–695.

Rahbar S, Figarola JL. 2003. Novel inhibitors of advanced glycation endproducts. *Archives of Biochemistry and Biophysics* 419: 63-79.

Ramu R, Prithvi S. Shirahatt , Farhan Zameer, Lakshmi V. Ranganatha, M.N. Nagendra Prasad. Inhibitory effect of banana (Musa sp. var. Nanjangud rasa bale) flower extract and its constituents Umbelliferone and Lupeol on α-glucosidase, aldose reductase and glycation at multiple stages. South African Journal of Botany 2014; 95: 54–63.

Rani M, Krishna MS, Padmakumari KP, Raghu KG, Sundaresan A. *Zingiber officinale* extract exhibits antidiabetic potential via modulating glucose uptake, protein glycation and inhibiting adipocyte differentiation: An *in vitro* study. *Science of Food Agriculture*. 2012; 92: 1948-1955.

Ratnasooriya WD, Walimuni KSM Abeysekera, Tharaka BS Muthunayake, Chatura DT Ratnasooriya. *In vitro* Antiglycation and Cross-Link Breaking Activities of Sri Lankan Low-Grown Orthodox Orange Pekoe Grade Black Tea (*Camellia sinensis* L). Tropical Journal of Pharmaceutical Research. 2014; 13(4): 567-571.

Rout S, Banerjee R. Free radical scavenging, anti-glycation and tyrosinase inhibition properties of a polysaccharide fraction isolated from the rind from *Punica granatum*. *Bioresource Technology* 2007; 98: 3159-3163.

Rutter K, Sell DR, Fraser N, Obrenovich M, Zito M, Starke-Reed P, Monnier VM. Green Tea Extract Suppresses the Age-Related Increase in Collagen Crosslinking and Fluorescent Products in C57BL/6 Mice. *International Journal for Vitamin and Nutrition Research*, 2003; 73(6): 453-460.

Singh P, Ramesha H. Jayaramaiah, Sachin B. Agawane, Garikapati Vannuruswamy, Arvind M. Korwar, Atul Anand, Vitthal S. Dhaygude, Mahemud L. Shaikh, Rakesh S. Joshi, Ramanamurthy Boppana, Mahesh J. Kulkarni, Hirekodathakallu V. Thulasiram, Ashok P. Giri. Potential Dual Role of Eugenol in Inhibiting Advanced Glycation End Products in Diabetes: Proteomic and Mechanistic Insights. Scientific Reports 2015; DOI: 10.1038/srep18798.

Singh R, Barden A, Mori T, Beilin L. Advanced glycation ednproducts: A review. *Diabetologia* 2001; 44: 129-146.

Soman S, Arun A. Rauf, Madambath Indira, Chellam Rajamanickam. Antioxidant and Antiglycative Potential of Ethyl Acetate Fraction of *Psidium guajava* Leaf Extract in Streptozotocin-Induced Diabetic Rats. Plant Foods Hum Nutr. 2010; 65: 386–391.

Suantawee T, Wesarachanon K, Anantsuphasak K, Daenphetploy T, Thienngern S, Thilavech T, Pasukamonset P, Ngamukote S, Adisakwattana S. Protein glycation inhibitory activity and antioxidant capacity of clove extract. Journal of Food Science and Technology. 2015; 52: 3843-3850.

Suzuki R, Miki Iijima, Yoshihito Okada,Toru Okuyama. Chemical Constituents of the Style of *Zea mays* L. with Glycation Inhibitory Activity. *Chem. Pharm. Bull.* 2007; 55(1): 153-155.

Trakoon-osot W, Uthai Sotanaphun, Pariya Phanachet, Supatra Porasuphatana, Umaporn Udomsubpayakul, Surat Komindr. Pilot study: Hypoglycemic and antiglycation activities of bitter melon (*Momordica charantia* L.) in type 2 diabetic patients. Journal of pharmacy research. 2013; 6: 859-864.

Tsuji-Naito K, Hiroshi Saeki, Miyuki Hamano. Inhibitory effects of *Chrysanthemum* species extracts on formation of advanced glycation end products. Food Chemistry 2009; 116: 854–859.

Wirasathien L, Pengsuparp T, Suttisri R *et al.* 2007. Inhibitors of aldose reductase and advanced glycation end products formation from the leaves of *Stelechocarpus cauliflorus. Phytomedicine* 14: 546-550.

Wu JW, Chiu-Lan Hsieh, Hsiao-Yun Wang, Hui-Yin Chen. Inhibitory effects of guava (*Psidium guajava* L.) leaf extracts and its active compounds on the glycation process of protein. Food Chemistry 2009; 113: 78–84.

Xiaofang Peng, Jinyu Ma, Feng Chen, Mingfu Wang. Naturally occurring inhibitors against the formation of advanced glycation end-products. Food Funct 2011; 2: 289–301.

Yamabe N, Kang KS, Goto E, Tanaka T, Yokozawa T. Beneficial effect of *Corni fructus*, a constituent of Hachimijio-gan, on advanced glycation end-productmediated renal injury in streptozotocin-treated diabetic rats. *Biological and Pharmaceutical Bulletin.* 2007a; 30: 520-526.

Yamabe N, Kang KS, Matsuo Y, Tanaka T, Yokozawa T. Identification of antidiabetic effect of iridoid glycosides and low molecular weight polyphenol fractions of *Corni fructus*, a constituent of hachimi-jio-gan, in streptozotocininduced diabetic rats. *Biological and Pharmaceutical Bulletin.* 2007b; 30: 1289-1296.

Yamaguchi F, Toshiaki Ariga, Yoshihiro Yoshimura, Hiroyuki Nakazawa. Antioxidative and Anti-Glycation Activity of Garcinol from *Garcinia indica* Fruit Rind. J. Agric. Food Chem. 2000; 48: 180-185.

Yang B, Mouming Zhao, Yueming Jiang. Anti-glycated activity of polysaccharides of longan (*Dimocarpus longan* Lour.) fruit pericarp treated by ultrasonic wave. Food Chemistry. 2009; 114: 629–633.

Yokozawa T, Akiko Satoh, Takako Nakagawa and Noriko Ya. Attenuating Effects of Wen-Pi-Tang Treatment in Rats with Diabetic Nephropathy. The American Journal of Chinese Medicine, 2006; 34: 307–321.

Yokozawa T, Kim HY, Cho EJ, Yamabi N, Choi JS. J. Protective effects of mustard leaf (*Brassica juncea*) against diabetic oxidative stress. Nutr. Sci. Vitaminol (Tokyo), 2003; 49: 87–93.

Yokozawa T, Takako Nakagawa T. Inhibitory effects of Luobuma tea and its components against glucose-mediated protein damage. Food and Chemical Toxicology 2004; 42: 975–981.

Yoshikawa M, Yutana Pongpiriyadacha, Akinobu Kishi, Tadashi Kageura, Tao Wang, Toshio Morikawa, Hisashi Matsuda. Biological Activities of *Salacia chinensis* originating in Thailand: The Quality Evaluation Guided by α-Glucosidase Inhibitory Activity. Yakugaku Zasshi. 2003; 123: 871–880.

Zielinska D, Dorota Szawara-Nowak, Henryk Zielinski. antioxidative and anti-glycation activity of buckwheat hull tea infusion. International Journal of Food Properties. 2013; 16:228–239.

Chapter 4

Plants used in the Management of Diabetic Complications

4.1 Introduction

Diabetes Mellitus (DM) is a chronic metabolic disorder of impaired metabolism of carbohydrates, fats and proteins, characterized by hyperglycemia resulting from decreased utilization of carbohydrate and excessive glycogenolysis and gluconeogenesis from amino acids and fatty acids (Pontiroli *et al.*, 1994). According to the recent reports, incidence of DM is about 6.4% globally affecting 285 million adults, in 2010 and will increase to 7.7%, affecting the 439 million adults by 2030 (Shaw *et al.*, 2010). People with DM are at higher risk of developing serious complications including heart attacks, blindness, kidney failure and neuropathy (Figure 4.1). Large prospective clinical studies show a strong relationship between glycaemia and diabetic micro vascular complications in DM (Nathan *et al.*, 1993). Four molecular mechanisms are being extensively studied for their role in causing diabetic complications; increase in the flux of glucose through polyol pathway, increased intracellular formation of advanced glycation end-products (AGEs), activation of protein kinase C (PKC) and increased flux through the hexosamine pathway (Brownlee 2001). Among these, polyol pathway plays an important role in the development of complications in DM (Gabbay 1973). Aldose reductase (AR) which is the first enzyme in the polyol pathway is a cytosolic, monomeric oxidoreductase enzyme that catalyses the NADPH-dependant reduction of glucose (Wilson et al., 1992). In the polyol pathway, sorbitol is oxidized to fructose by the enzyme sorbitol dehydrogenase, with NAD^+ reduced to NADH. Hyperglycemia induced polyol flux leads to increase in sorbitol induced osmotic stress, decreased $(Na^+$ & $K^+)$ ATP ase activity, an increase in cytosolic $NADH/NAD^+$ ratio and a decrease in cytosolic NADPH. As NADPH is required for regenerating reduced glutathione (GSH), this could induce or exacerbate intracellular oxidative stress leading to changes in respiration, membrane metabolism, and oxidative resistance (Garcia *et al.,* 2001; Lee *et al.,* 1999). Since it is not possible to demonstrate a derived factor of ARI activity that has more prognostic value for diabetic complications, a critical review of the literature on various aldose reductase inhibitors (ARIs) from plants and their actual mechanism by which they produce a beneficial effect on progression of diabetic complications has been studied.

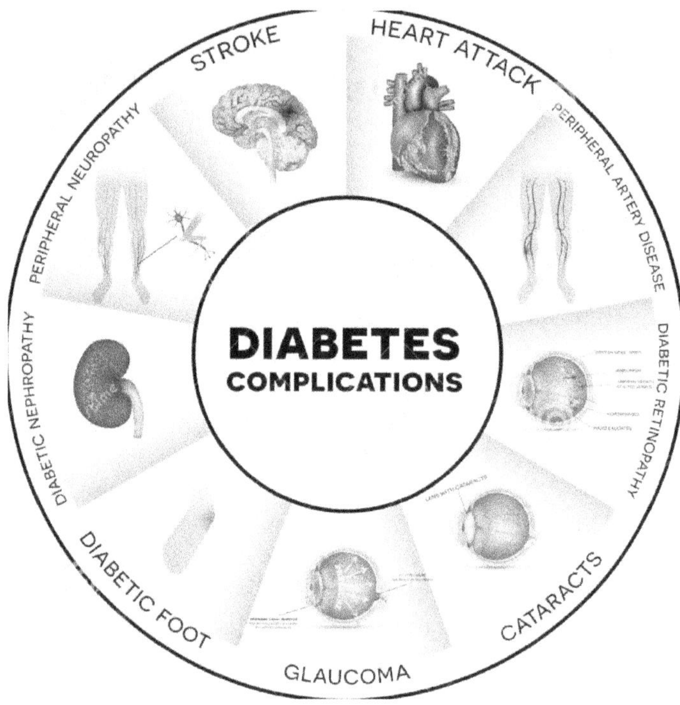

Figure 4.1 Download from google.com. (Diabetes Complications Stock Illustration - Image: 62541059)

Even though, a large variety of compounds have been synthesized with potent *in vitro* aldose reductase inhibitory (ARI) activity, very few compounds are clinically available because of undesirable side effects and poor pharmacokinetics (Rosenstock et al., 1987). The failure of these compounds has increased the need for search of newer molecules from natural sources. Till date numerous plant extracts and their phytoconstituents have been reported to have aldose reductase activity, phytoconstituents with ARI property which studied in diabetic Complications shown in figure 4.2, but a specific book on the efficacy of these ARIs in the management of various diabetic complications has not yet been published. The present book aims at critical appraisal of the available literature on various ARIs from plants for their role in the management of diabetic complications.

Figure 4.2 phytoconstituents with ARI property which studied in diabetic complications.

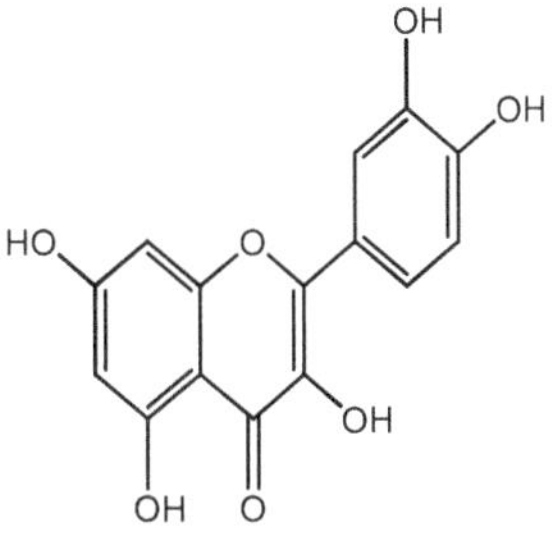

1

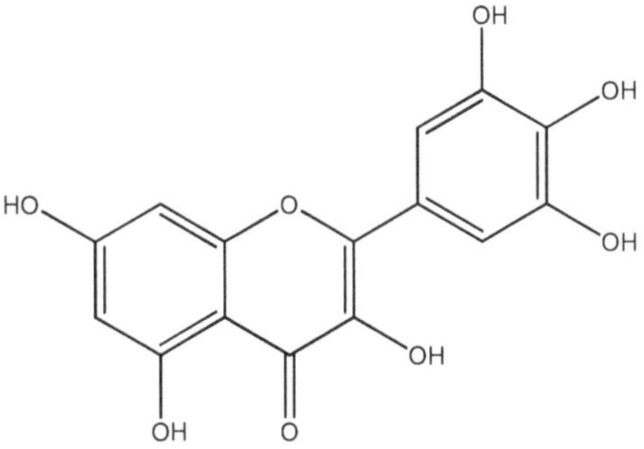

2

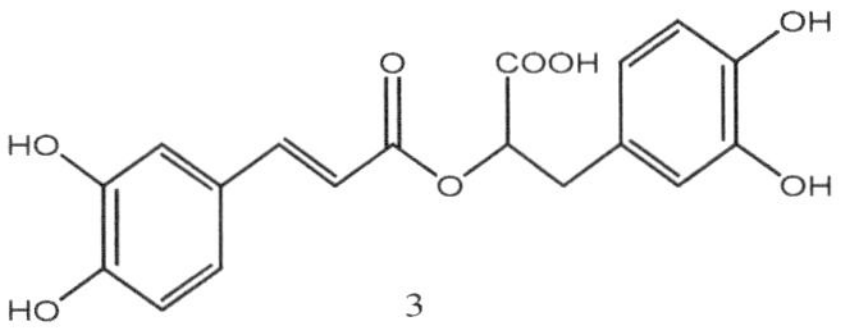

3

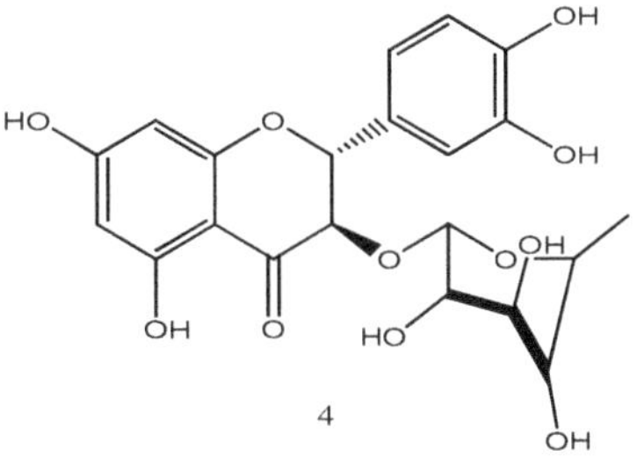

4

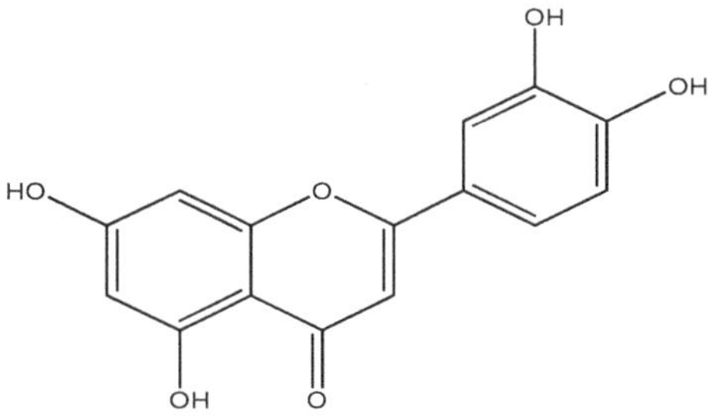

5

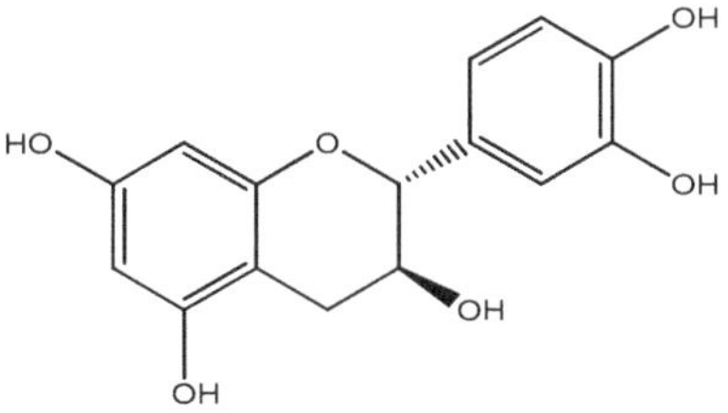

6

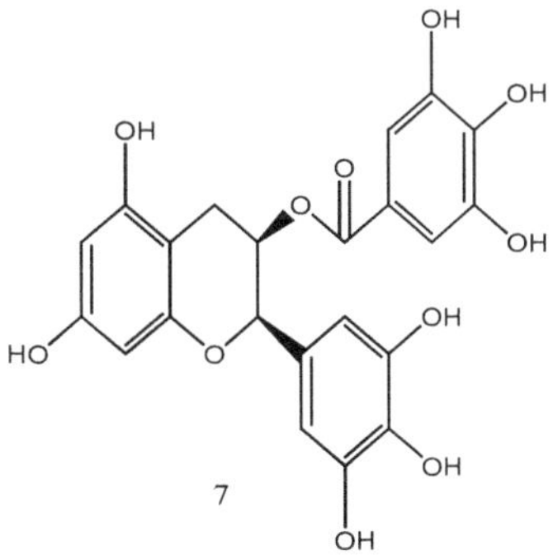

7

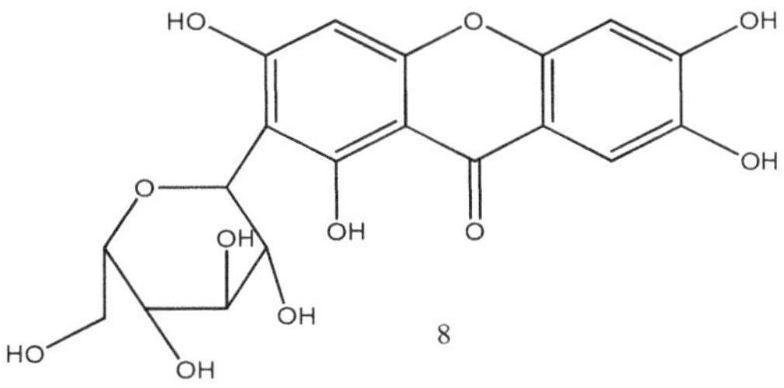

8

Figure 4.2 *Contd....*

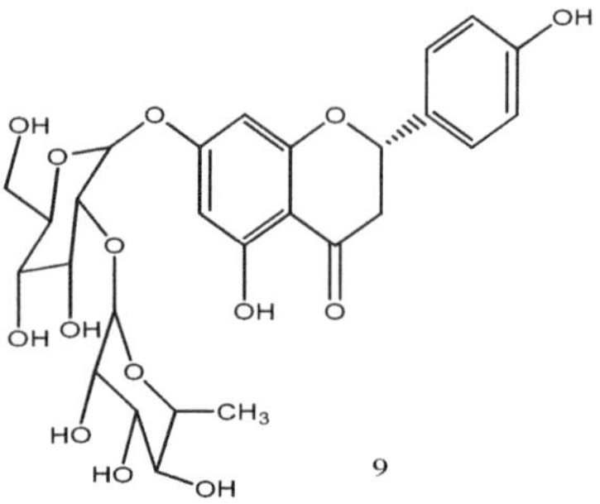

Figure 4.2 *Contd....*

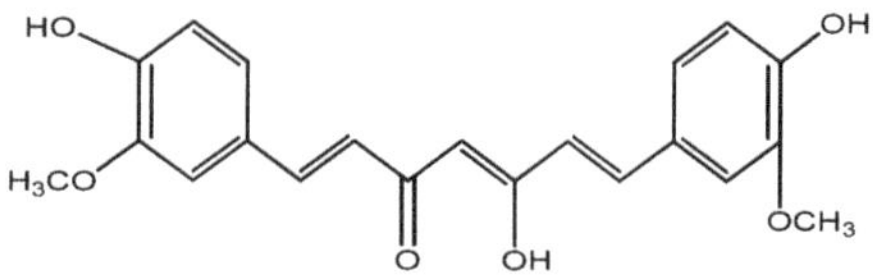

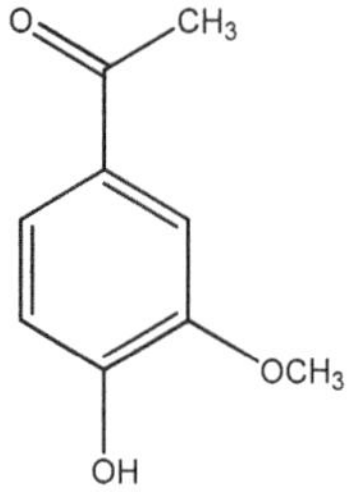

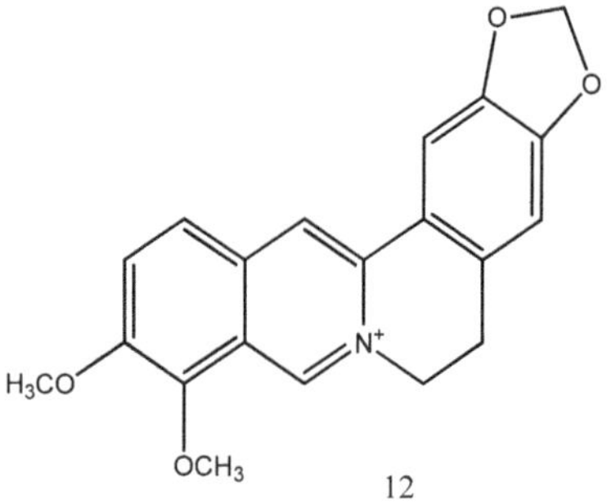

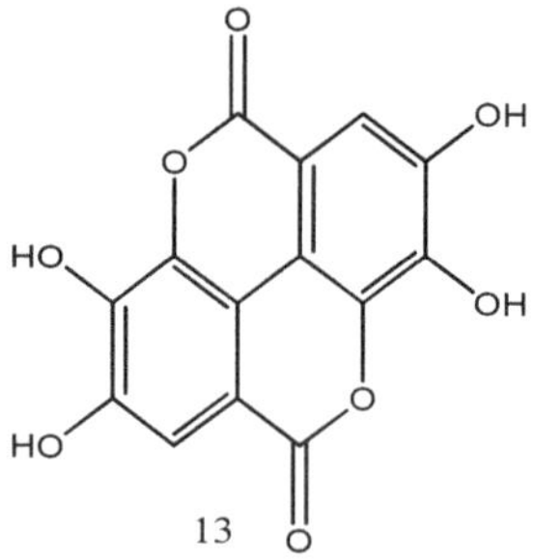

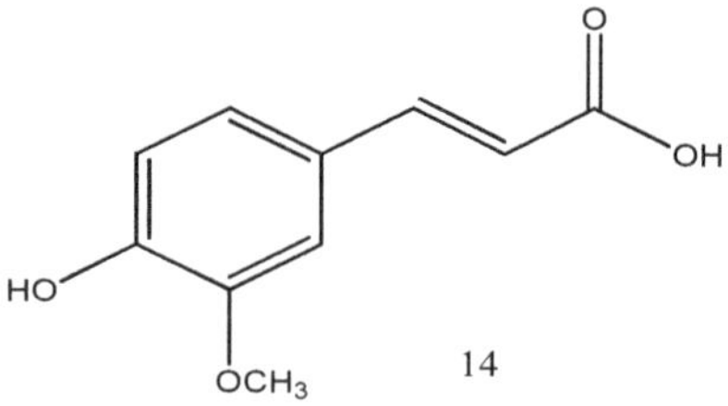

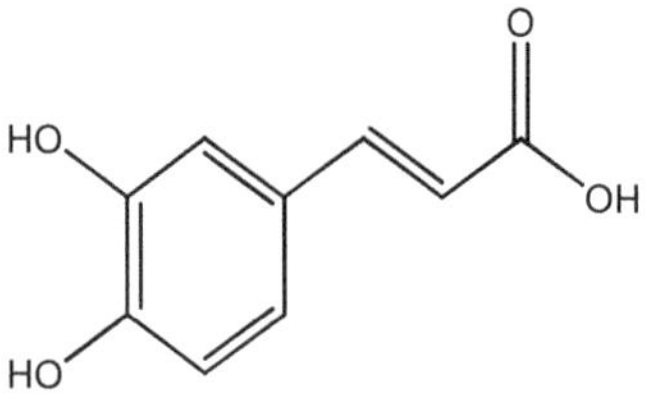

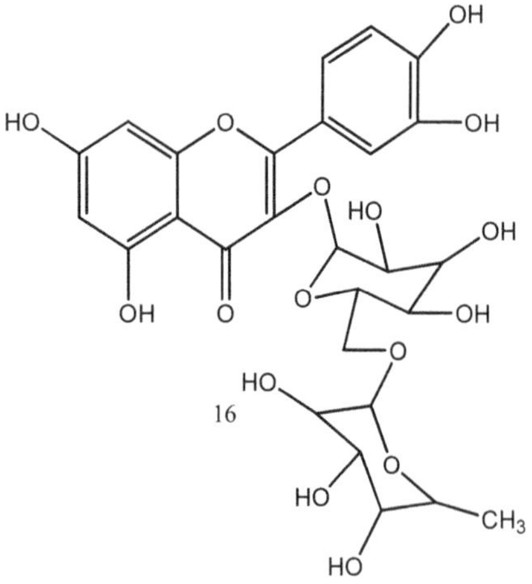

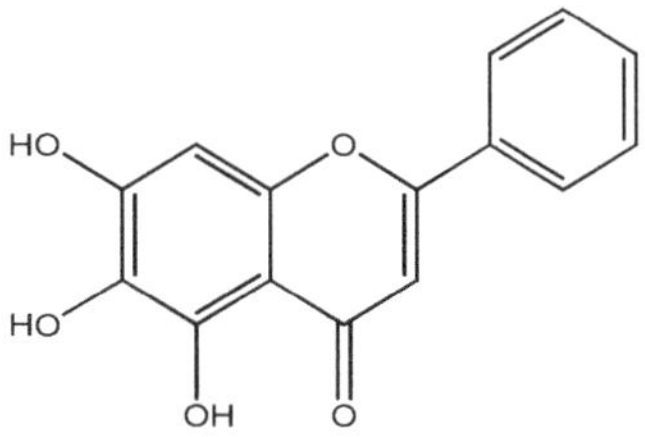

Figure 4.2 Contd....

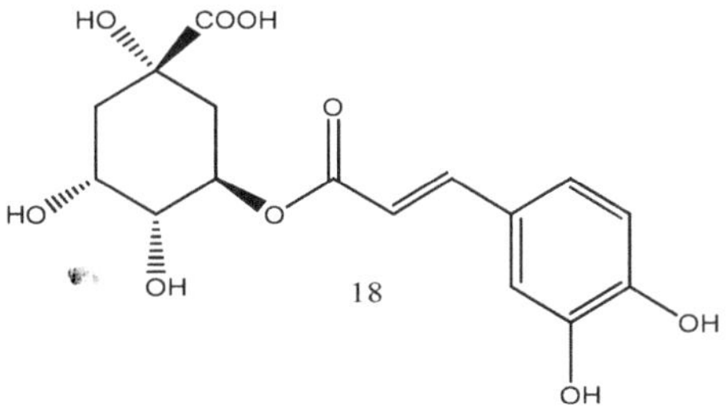

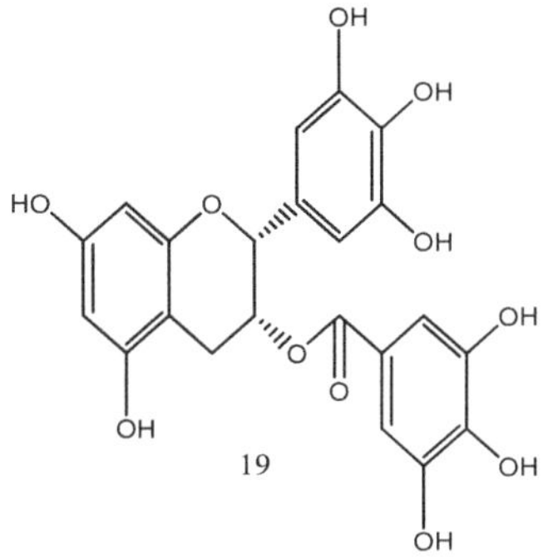

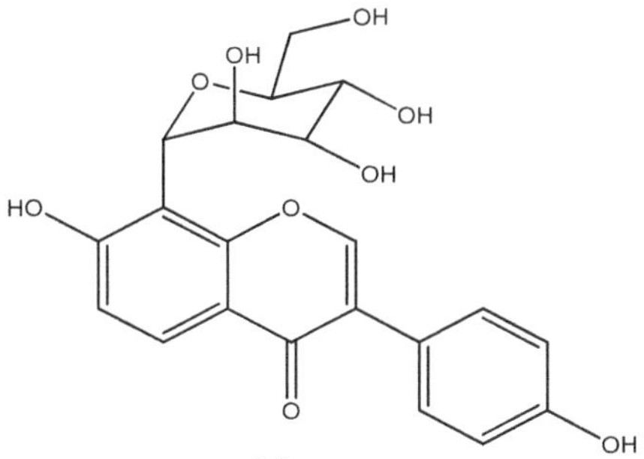

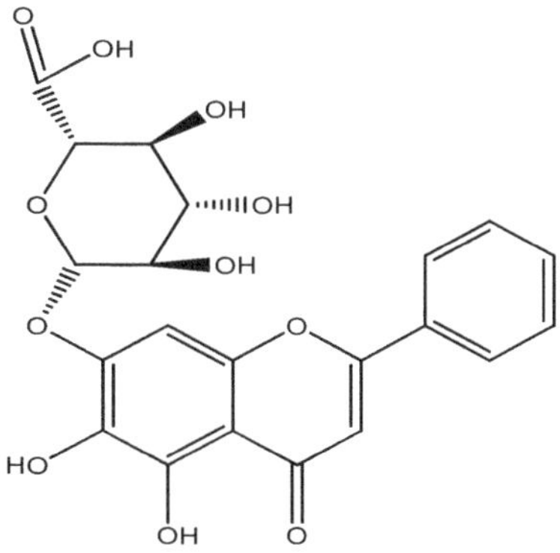

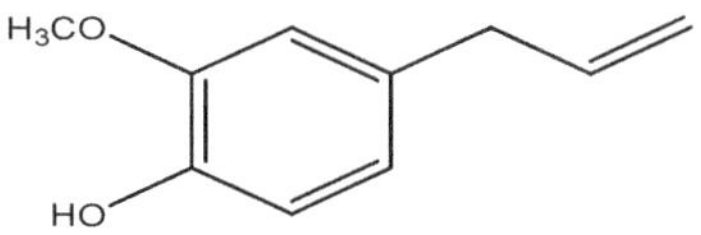

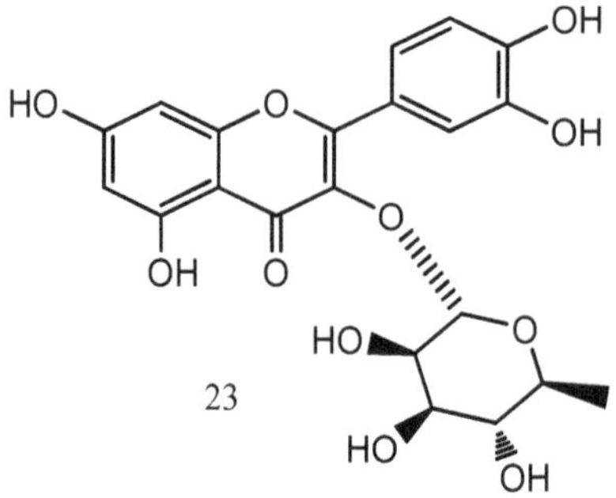

23

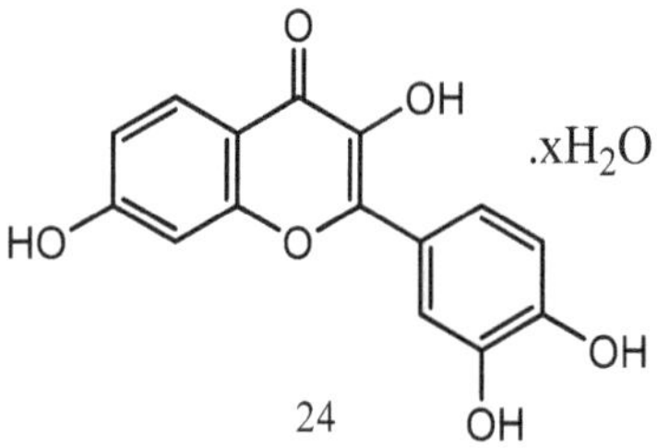

.xH$_2$O

24

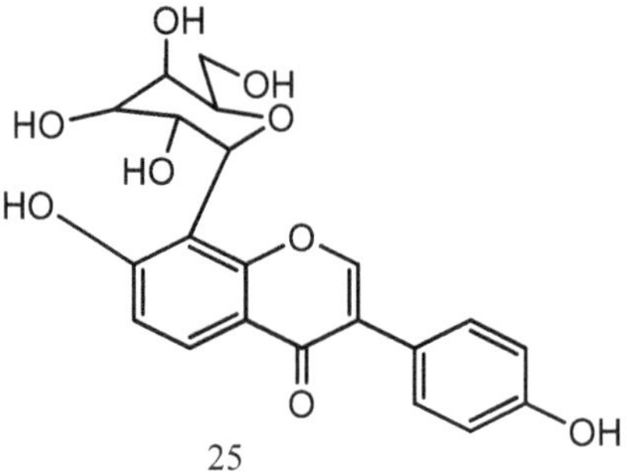

25

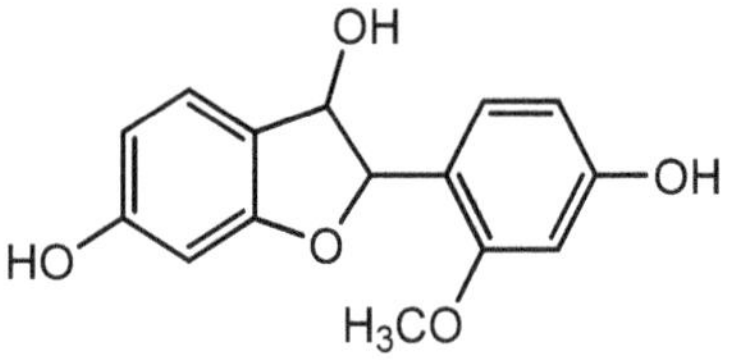

26

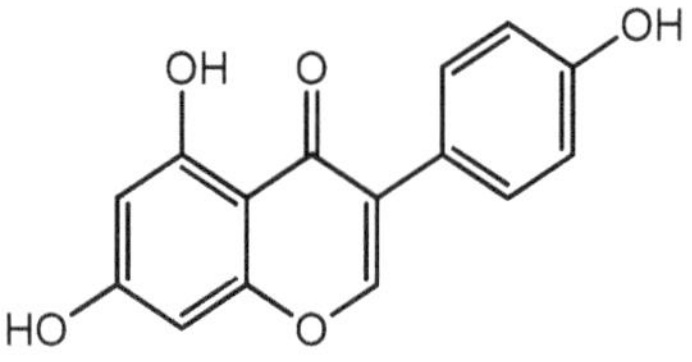

27

Diabetic Nephropathy

Diabetic nephropathy or diabetic kidney disease is one of the most important complications and affects 20-30 % of patients with DM. It is a progressive condition culminating into a kidney failure. Diabetic nephropathy has been classically defined by the presence of proteinuria greater than 0.5g/24h. The onset of diabetic nephropathy was found to be 17 years after the diagnosis of DM (Krolewski *et al.*, 1985). The pathogenic role of AR in diabetic nephropathy is a significant increase of the enzyme in the glomerulus (Kasajima *et al.*, 2001). Hyperactivation of AR in renal cells leads to the generation of AGEs. These AGEs along with the generation of reactive oxygen species (ROS) results in the expression and activation of transcription factors like nuclear factor NF-κB and PKC which are implicated in the pathogenesis of diabetic nephropathy (Figure 4.3).

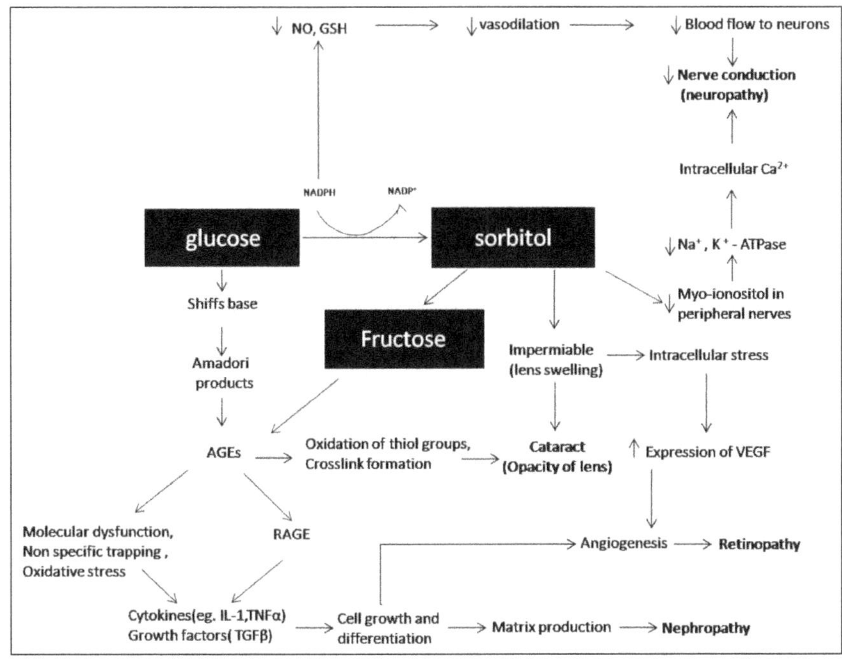

Figure 4.3 Flow diagram illustrating interplay between the polyol pathway, oxidative stress and diabetic complications. (Dodda *et al.*, 2014).

AGEs also contribute to the release of pro inflammatory cytokines, expression of growth factors and adhesion molecules (Kapor-Drezgic *et al.*, 1999; Oates *et al.*, 1999). This data suggests that inhibition of AR in kidney contributes to the protective effect on diabetic kidney.

Flavonoids like quercetin and myricetin which were reported to have potent ARI activity were found to show protective effect as well as prophylactic role on the diabetic kidney by decreasing the oxidative stress (Varma *et al.*, 1975; Anjaneyulu *et al.*, 2004; Ozcan *et al.*, 2012). In different studies, rosmarinic acid isolated from *Origanum vulgare,* nepetrin and nepetin isolated from *Rosmarinus officinalis* showed potent ARI activity. The aqueous extract of leaves of *R. officinalis* was found to alleviate the nephrotoxicity induced by CCl_4 in albino rats which was attributed to the antioxidative activity of one or more of its constituents. However, administration of rosmarinic acid alone was reported to inhibit glomerular hypertrophy, reduce glomerulosclerosis significantly in diabetic rats (Tomás-Barberán *et al.*, 1986; Koukoulitsa *et al.*, 2006; Majid *et al.*, 2011; Saber *et al.*, 2012).

Haraguchi *et al.*, (1996) investigated the ARI activity of isoquircetin and other flavonoids isolated from *Polygonun hydropiper*. In another study by Li *et al.*, (2011) isoquercetrin was found to display a strong scavenging ability for nitrite and nitric oxide (NO) and exhibited a protective effect on the kidneys of mice. Moreover, isoquercetin can increase the superoxide dimutase or catalase activities and reduce the manoldialdehyde, protein carbonyl and NO levels in the livers and kidneys of mice.

The dihydroflavonol astilbin isolated from the leaves of *Englhardtia chrysolepis* has been reported to show ARI activity whereas astilbin isolated from the rhizome of *Smilax china* L significantly ameliorates diabetic nephropathy by reducing renal production of transforming growth factor (TGF) -β1 and connective tissue growth factor (Haraguchi *et al.*, 1997; Chen *et al.*, 2011). The ARI activity of components isolated from active fractions of *Chrysanthemum indicum* have been examined and among the tested compounds, luteolin was found to show potent ARI activity, which was found to prevent morphological destruction of kidney in diabetic rats caused by increased oxidative stress induced by polyol pathway. One of the mechanisms of the renoprotective effect of luteolin was also related to increasing heme oxygenase-1 expression and elevating antioxidant status in diabetic nephropathy (Yoshikawa *et al.*, 1999; Wang *et al.*, 2011).

Murata *et al.*, (1994) reported the inhibitory activity of various phytoconstituents isolated from green tea which showed varying degrees of ARI effect with (-)-epigallocatechin having no activity. These catechins composing epigallocatechin, epicatechin gallate and epicatechin were found to normalize the morphological alterations in diabetic rats, indicating that catechin has renoprotective effects on diabetic nephropathy (Hase *et al.*, 2006). Yamabe *et al.*, 2006 reported the beneficial effect of (-)-epigallocatechin 3-O-gallate on diabetic nephropathy via suppressing hyperglycemia, AGEs, their related oxidative stress and cytokine activations, and there by altering the pathological states due to its multifocal mechanisms.

Phytochemical analysis of *Salacia chinensis* led to the isolation of mangiferin which was found to be a potent ARI (Morikawa *et al.*, 2003). Mangiferin improved the renal function in diabetic rats, which was manifested by its decreasing effect on 24 h urinary albumin excretion. This beneficial effect was related to mangiferin's inhibitory effect on over expression of TGF-β1, AGE and extra cellular matrix accumulation, polyol pathway activation, ROS generation and mesangial cells proliferation (Li *et al.*, 2010).

Goodarzi *et al.*, (2006) investigated the ARI effect of naringin in streptozotocin (STZ) induced diabetic rats. It was found that the inhibitory effect of naringin was comparable to that of quercetin. Besides this, naringin prevented the pathological alterations due to its insulin-sensitizing, anti-inflammatory, anti-dyslipidaemic and antioxidant activity. The mechanism for such an outcome is modulation of PPARγ, and NF-kB protein expression by naringin in kidney tissue indicating that naringin is an effective therapeutic strategy for the treatment of DM and its associated complications (Sharma *et al.*, 2011).

Curcumin, a potent inhibitor of AR was reported to show its efficacy in diabetic nephropathy. It reverses the alterations in the activities of kidney cellular enzymes associated with DM, reverses the decrease in polyunsaturated fatty acids to saturated fatty acids ratio and ATPases activity of renal membranes, and lowers nephromegaly in diabetic animals. Curcumin also acts through prevention of nuclear translocation of NF-kB which is responsible for mesangial expansion (Du *et al.*, 2006; Suresh *et al.*, 1998; Chiu *et al.*, 2009).

Nine isoflavonoids isolated from *Belamcanda chinensis* showed varying degrees of ARI activity. Even though there are no reports on the protective effect of the plant on diabetic nephropathy, apocynin, one of the constituent of the plant with NADPH oxidase inhibitory activity was found to block the effect of increased glucose concentration to activate PKC-induced NADPH oxidase, and fibronectin secretion by peritoneal cells. Apocynin blocks the increase in PKC, O^{-2} generation and proliferation during incubation of mesangial cells with glycated albumin (Jung *et al.*, 2002; Asaba *et al.*, 2005).

Ellagic acid isolated from *Myrciaria dubia* and caffeic acid isolated from *Origanum vulgare* were found to be inhibit AR *in vitro* and was also found to significantly diminish renal activity of aldose reductase and sorbitol dehydrogenase, as well as suppressed renal aldose reductase mRNA expression along with inhibition of IL-6, IL-1β, tumor necrosis factor (TNF)-α and monocyte chemoattractant protein 1 *in vivo* suggesting the combined effect of ARI and anti-inflammatory activities of ellagic acid for its beneficial role in diabetic nephropathy (Ueda *et al.*, 2004; Chao *et al.*, 2010).

Kato *et al.* (2006) investigated the ARI activity of various phytoconstituents in rhizome of *Zingiber officinalis* Roscoe was found to posses' good inhibitory activity. However, the protective effect of the plant on diabetic kidney was characterized by the inhibition of structural distortions that developed by increased free radicals after a short period of hyper glycaemia. Besides this the plant was found to protect the kidney against the endothelial dysfunction resulting from membranous glycation (Qattan *et al.*, 2008). Chethan *et al.* (2008) reported the AR inhibiting activity of ferulic acid and other constituents isolated from Finger millet (*Eleusine coracana*) were found to show renal protective effects through improved glycemic control and renal structural changes, which are involved in the inhibition of oxidative stress, inflammation and the expression of TGF-β1 and type IV collagen (Choi *et al.*, 2011).

Butein isolated from bark of *Rhus verniciflua* was found to be a potent inhibitor of HRAR but the nephroprotective activity of the compound was attributed to its antioxidant ability and also the renal concentrating ability (Lee *et al.*, 2008; Kang *et al.*, 2004). Berberine isolated from *Coptis japonica* was found to possess potent ARI activity, also showed the renoprotective effects which was related to inhibition of glycosylation and improvement of antioxidation leading to upregulation of renal nephrin and podocin expressions (Lee 2002; Wu *et al.*, 2012) (Table 4.1).

Table 4.1 Phytochemical with ARI property which were studied in diabetic nephropathy. (Dodda *et al.*, 2014)

Compound	Mechanism of action
Quercetin (1)	Reducing the oxidative stress
Myricetin (2)	Reducing the oxidative stress
Rosmarinic Acid (3)	Reducing the oxidative stress
Astilbin (4)	Inhibition of inflammatory mediators.
Luteloin (5)	Reducing the oxidative stress
Catechin (6)	Reducing the oxidative stress
( )-Epigallocatechin 3-O-Gallate (7)	Decreased AGEs induced oxidative stress, anti inflammatory property.
Mangiferin (8)	Decreased AGEs induced oxidative stress, anti inflammatory property.
Naringin (9)	Antioxidant and anti-inflammatory property
Curcumin (10)	Cholesterol lowering ability
Apocynin (11)	Decreased PKC. Decreased oxidative stress,
Berberine (12)	Decreased AGEs and decreased oxidative stress
Ellagic Acid (13)	Decreased AR, glycative and inflammatory mediators
Ferulic acid (14)	Antioxidant and anti-inflammatory property
Caffeic acid (15)	Decreased AR, glycative and inflammatory mediators

Even though inhibition of AR plays a considerable role in the development of diabetic nephropathy, experimental studies with ARI in animal models in various studies have produced remarkably contradictory results. Treatment with tolrestat reduced the progression of urinary albumin excretion when compared to diabetic control rats whereas other studies have failed to show this protective effect. Some studies have reported the normalization of tissue sorbitol without much effect on urinary albumin excretion. Similarly, glomerular filtration rate was found to be normalized in some studies while others have failed to show this effect on glomerular filtration rate (Boel *et al.*, 1995). Apart from these, various studies on AR inhibitors shown their efficacy in diabetic nephropathy with mechanisms like decrease in oxidative stress induced damage, anti-inflammatory effect etc. which infers that even some of the potent AR inhibitors like quercetin were found to reduce the oxidative damage that may be caused by activation of AR or by any other mechanisms. Thus, in this situation, it can be concluded that, a multiple therapy which aims at different causative factors and various mechanisms rather than AR alone would be more beneficial in the therapy and prevention of diabetic nephropathy.

Diabetic Neuropathy

Neuropathy is a common complication of both type 1 and type 2 DM with a prevalence of about 8% in newly diagnosed individuals to 50% in patients with long standing disease. There are many different diabetic neuropathies involving different nerve types which are mainly characterized by diffuse or focal damage to peripheral somatic or autonomic nerve fibers resulting from DM. Diabetic neuropathy can be classified into diffuse and focal neuropathies with diffuse neuropathy being more common, chronic and progressive where as focal neuropathies are less common and acute in nature. However, all these neuropathies are thought to occur from hyperglycemia induced damage to nerve cells and from neuronal ischemia resulting from hyperglycemia induced changes in the four pathways described above (Edwards *et al.*, 2008).

Increase in sorbitol concentrations by polyol pathway leads to cellular injury and decrease of *myo*-ionositol in the peripheral nerves and thereby leading to decrease in Na^+/K^+ - ATPase activity which is essential for nerve conduction (Oka *et al.*, 2001). Moreover, decreased NADPH results in decreased NO and reduced GSH production resulting in decreased vasodilatation and increased ROS production and oxidative damage (Figure 3). Thus, AR inhibitors are likely to contribute to the beneficial effect on development of diabetic neuropathy. A detailed of reports on AR inhibitors from medicinal plants showing their effect on neuropathy and their mechanism has been described (Table 4.2). Advantages and limitations of some selective animal models of diabetic neuropathy developed since 1960s are summarized in table 4.3.

Table 4.2 Phytochemical with ARI property which were studied in diabetic neuropathy. (Dodda *et al.*, 2014)

Compound	Mechanism of action
Quercetin (1)	Central analgesic activity
Rutin (16)	Metal chelating property
Baicalein (17)	Anti oxidative, anti inflammatory and inhibition of sorbitol pathway

Table 4.2 *Contd...*

Compound	Mechanism of action
Chlorogenic acid (18)	Anti-oxidative and anti-inflammatory properties
Epigallocatechin-gallate (19)	Antioxidant property
Ellagic acid (13)	Antioxidant property
Naringin (9)	Antioxidant property
Curcumin (10)	Anti-oxidative and anti-inflammatory properties
Puerarin (20)	Dilation of blood vessels (no exact mechanism)
Baicalin (21)	Inhibition of AR
Eugenol (22)	NO mediated vasodilatation

Table 4.3 Advantages and limitations of some selective animal models of diabetic neuropathy developed since 1960s. (Shahidul *et al.*, 2013).

Animals models	Characterization of diabetic neuropathy/advantages	Limitations
Streptozotocin-induced rat model (classic)	1. Reduced sizes of nerve fiber, axon, and myelin sheath. 2. Impaired motor function	Not validated by antineuropathic drug.
Streptozotocin induced rat model (recent)	1. Significantly reduced right and left fascicular areas and myelination of phrenic nerves. 2. Validated by insulin (s.c.).	1. Some major pathogenesis of diabetic neuropathy has not been characterized. 2. Although validated by insulin (s.c.), no antineuropathic drug has been used.
C57BL/Ks (db/db) mice model (classic)	1. Severely decreased motor nerve conduction velocity (MNCV). 2. Absence of large myelinated fibers. 3. Axonal atrophy. 4. Axonal dystrophy in myelinated and unmyelinated fibers. 5. Loss, shrinkage, and breakdown of myeline sheath.	Not evaluated by any antidiabetic or antineuropathic drug.
Genetically modified C57BL/Ks (db/db) mice model (recent)	1. Increased body weight, hyperglycemia, and hyperlipidemia. 2. Lower tail flick response to heat stimulus, sciatic motor nerve conduction velocity, and intraepididymal nerve fiber velocity.	1. Mismatched results were observed for body weight, blood glucose, plasma lipids, and blood glycated hemoglobin. 2. Not validated by anti-diabetic or antineuropathic drugs.

Table 4.3 *Contd...*

Animals models	Characterization of diabetic neuropathy/advantages	Limitations
Streptozotocin induced C57BL6/J mice model	1. Peroxynitrite injury in peripheral nerve and dorsal root ganglion neurons. 2. Motor and sensory nerve conduction velocity deficits, thermal and mechanical hyperplasia, tactile allodynia, and loss of intraepidermal nerve fibers.	Not validated by using antineuropathic drug.
Streptozotoc ininduced Diabetic sensory neuropathic ddYmice model	1. Significantly lower sensory nerve conduction velocity, higher nociceptive threshold, hypoalgesia, and unmyelinated fiber atrophy. 2. Successfully evaluated by insulin treatment. 3. Can be a better model to study the human sensory polyneuropathy.	No significant change was found in the myelinated nerve fiber areas.
Chinese hamster neuropathic model	Reduced conduction velocity of both motor and sensory components of hind lamb nerves (16–22%).	1. Peripheral diabetic neuropathy (PDN) was less severe than human diabetic neuropathy. 2. Further study needed for proper validation.
Rhesus monkey model of PDN	1. Significantly reduced motor conduction velocity. 2. Prolonged F-wave latencies. 3. Pathogeneses' resembles to humans.	1. No difference in motor-evoked amplitudes. 2. Prolonged nerve conduction induction time (2 years). 3. Not validated by antineuropathic drug.
Spontaneously diabetic WBN/Kob rat model	1. Slower motor nerve conduction and temporal dispersion of compound muscle action potential. 2. Structural de- and remyelination in the sciatic and tibial nerves at 12 month. 3. Axonal degeneration, dystrophy, and reduced myelinated fiber at 20 month. 4. Resembles human pathogenesis of PDN.	Not validated by antineuropathic drug.
L-fucose induced neuropathic rat model	1. Reduced Na+-K+-ATPase activity. 2. Reduced nerve conduction velocity. 3. Axonal dystrophy. 4. Paranodal swelling and demyelination without increasingWalleran degeneration of nerve fiber loss.	Not validated by antineuropathic drug.

Table 4.3 *Contd...*

Animals models	Characterization of diabetic neuropathy/advantages	Limitations
Partial sciatic nerve ligated rat model	1. Produced long-lasting mechanical, but thermal hyperalgesia. 2. Evaluated by ant-diabetic neuropathic drugs.	Major pathogenesis was not characterized.
Nonobese diabetic (NOD) mice model	1. Short induction period. 2. Markedly swollen axons and dendrites (neurotic dystrophy). 3. Consistent with the pathogenesis of other rodent models of PDN and human PDN. 4. Suggested as a better model than ICR mice particularly in terms of nerve regeneration.	Not validated by antineuropathic drug.
Spontaneously induced Ins2 Akita mouse model	1. Spontaneously induced diabetic model. 2. Progressive and sustained chronic hyperglycemia. 3. Reduced sensory nerve conduction velocity. 4. Markedly swollen axons and dendrites (neurotic dystrophy). 5. Consistent with the pathogenesis of other rodent models of PDN and human PDN.	Not validated by anti-diabetic or antineuropathic drug.
Leptin-deficient (ob/ob) mice model	1. Clearly manifested thermal hypoalgesia. 2. Relatively higher nonfasting blood glucose level (20mmol/L). 3. Slow motor and sensory nerve conduction. 4. Significant reduction of intraepidermal nerve fiber. 5. Validated by antiperipheral diabetic neuropathic drug.	May not be widely available for routine pharmacological screening of anti-diabetic or anti-neuropathic drugs.
Otsuka Long-Evans Tokushima Fatty (OLETF) rats model	1. Significantly higher blood glucose and HbA1c levels. 2. Reduced motor nerve conduction velocity and thermal nociception.	1. Some major pathogenesis of PDN has not been characterized. 2. Not validated by anti-diabetic neuropathic drugs.
Rat insulin I promoter/human interferon-beta (RIP/IFNβ) transgenic ICR mice model	1. Significantly hyperglycemia, slower tibial sensory nerve conduction velocity. 2. Reduced nerve fiber density and increased motor latencies.	1. A sophisticated surgical approach has been used to develop the model. 2. Not validated by anti-diabetic or antineuropathic drugs.

Table 4.3 *Contd...*

Animals models	Characterization of diabetic neuropathy/advantages	Limitations
High-fat diet-fed female C57BL6/J mice model	1. Deficit of motor and sensory nerve conductions, tactile allodynia, and thermal hypoalgesia. 2. Can be used as model for prediabetic or obesity related neuropathy.	1. Intradermal nerve fiber loss, and axonal atrophy was absent. 2. Cannot be used for chronic diabetic neuropathy. 3. Not validated by antineuropathic drugs.
Surgically induced neuropathic model	1. Thermal and mechanical hyperalgesia in paw and tail. 2. Reduced nerve fiber density and nerve Conduction velocity. 3. Very short induction period.	1. Not validated by using antineuropathic drug. 2. Not suitable to study the human diabetic neuropathy.
Genetically modified SDT fatty rat model	1. Sustained hyperglycemia and dyslipidemia with delayed and reduced motor nerve Conduction velocity. 2. Lower number of sural nerve fibers and Thickened epinural arterioles. 3. Successfully validated by anti-diabetic Drug such as pioglitazone.	Some pathogenesis was induced only after a long period of time such as 40 Weeks.

A potent natural AR inhibitor quercetin was found to increase nociceptive threshold indicating an antinociceptive activity of quercetin in diabetic rats (Anjaneyulu *et al.*, 2003). However, quercetin affecting the physiological and biochemical alterations leading to diabetic neuropathy was not yet reported. Another AR inhibitor rutin was found to show a protective effect against diabetic neuropathy by its metal chelating property. It was proposed to sequester the transition metal preventing the fenton reaction which may contribute to the development of diabetic neuropathy (Je *et al.*, 2002). The protective effect of baicalein was attributed to various mechanisms like inhibition of PKC, oxidative stress and LOX pathways but do not sorbitol pathway even though the compound was reported to be a potent AR inhibitor (Stavniichuk *et al.*, 2011). A phenolic AR inhibitor chlorogenic acid was found to show antihyperalgesic activity due to its antioxidant and anti-inflammatory properties (Bagdas *et al.*, 2012). Similarly, the beneficial effect of a potent AR inhibitor epigallocatechin-gallate against diabetic neuropathy was due to the inhibition of oxidative stress in diabetic rats (Tourandokht et al., 2012).

Ellagic acid which is a potent AR inhibitor along with antioxidant property was found to show a protective effect against diabetic neuropathy by its antioxidant property. It was found to significantly decrease MDA and nitrate levels in diabetic rats when compared to control group (Uzar *et al.*,

2012). Likewise, a potent antioxidant, naringin with a ARI property was found to exhibit neuroprotective effect in diabetic rats by down regulation of free radical and cytokine regulated TNF-α (Kandhare *et al.,* 2012). Similarly, an isoflavonoid, puerarin was found to increase the conductive velocity of the nerves which is due to the dilation of blood vessels leading to improvement of micro circulation and reduced blood viscosity. However, the mechanism by which these alterations occurred were yet to be studied (Xie *et al.,* 1998). Chronic treatment with curcumin, a potent AR inhibitor and antioxidant led to inhibition of NO and TNF- α and there by antihyperalgesic activity in diabetic rats (Sharma *et al.,* 2006).

Baicalin was found to show a protective effect and relieve clinical symptoms of diabetic neuropathy by direct inhibition of AR in diabetic rats (Yanhu *et al.,* 1999). Similarly, eugenol, a potent AR inhibitor was found to improve diabetic neuropathy by augmentation of NO and endothelium-derived hyperpolarising factor (EDHF) - mediated vasorelaxation (Nangle *et al.,* 2006).

Aremisia dracunculus, a plant with various potent ARIs exhibited a beneficial effect of diabetic neuropathy by decreasing the sciatic nerve and spinal cord 12/15-lipoxygenase activation and oxidative nitrosative stress but has failed to ameliorate hyperglycemia or reduce sciatic nerve sorbitol pathway (Logendra *et al.,* 2006; Watcho *et al.,* 2011). Likewise, the curative and preventive property of Trigonella in diabetic neuropathy was due to improvement in glucose intolerance, anti-inflammatory and antioxidant property even though the plant was found to possess a potent ARI activity (Nanjundan *et al.,* 2009; Saraswat *et al.,* 2008).

Administration of a *Momordica charantia* with a potent ARI activity in diabetic rats led to a slight increase in myelinated fiber area. Even though, the mechanism for this beneficial effect of *M. charantia* administration on the structural abnormalities of peripheral nerves in experimental DM was not established, however, the antioxidative property of the plant for the prevention of functional abnormalities in STZ-diabetic rats (Celia *et al.,* 2003).

Apart from the above mentioned, plants such as *Olea europaea* with no reported AR activity was found to be effective against diabetic neuropathy and was found to attenuate thermal hyperalgesia in diabetic rats. The plant was found to show the effect by preventing the glucose induced neuronal apoptosis (Kaeidi *et al.,* 2011).

Diabetic Cataract

Cataract is a condition where the crystalline lens of the eye loses its transparency. DM has been associated with an increase in cataract among adults (Ederer *et al.,* 1981). Cataract in DM is mainly caused by swelling of crystalline lens due to osmotic changes caused by increased sorbitol concentration. The other mechanism is the cross linking of lens proteins due to non enzymatic glycosylation. These glycated products generally called as AGEs readily accumulate in the lens and cause oxidation of thiol groups, cross link formation and aggregation of the crystalline proteins producing high molecular weight insoluble proteins which are responsible for opacification (Ahmed 2005) (Figure 4.3). Thus, the polyol pathway plays a momentous role in the formation of cataract in DM.

Even though various classes of drugs such as antioxidants, vitamins, NSAIDs, etc. have been developed which aim to interact with the altered lens metabolism in cataract, ARIs remain to be the most studied class of drugs. The role of these drugs in the prevention of diabetic cataract is now well established and various natural and synthetic ARIs are under active research. A good number of synthetic compounds have been found to exhibit anticataract potential in different animal models and clinical trials. Nevertheless, even various natural compounds were found to possess good anticataract activity (Table 4.4-4.5). Thus, here briefly explain of various herbal ARIs and their mechanism in inhibiting the diabetic cataract has been compiled.

To date numerous studies were conducted to evaluate the anticataract activity of different medicinal plants and phytoconstituents. Enlisting a few of them, green tea was found to inhibit AR, glycated protein and along with its hypoglycemic affect, it was found to show anticataract activity in diabetic rats (Joe *et al.*, 2005). Similarly, *Adhatoda vasica* exhibited anticataract activity by inhibiting lens AR. Administration of byakangelicin to diabetic rats led to of suppression of sorbitol leading to increase in Na^+/K^+ ATPase and thereby exhibiting a protective effect on diabetic cataract. However, the mechanism was not proposed. *Trigonella foenum-graceum* and *Pterocarpus marsupium* were found to exhibit anticataract activity by means of antihyperglycemic effect with trigonella exhibiting ARI activity while there is no ARI activity reported for the later (Saraswat *et al.*, 2008; Gacche *et al.,* 2011) (Table 4.4).

Table 4.4 Plants with ARI property which were studied in diabetic cataract. (Dodda *et al.*, 2014)

Plant	Type of cataract	Mechanism of action
Pterocarpus marsupium	Diabetic cataract	Anti hyperglycemic affect
Trigonella foenum-graecum	Diabetic cataract	Anti hyperglycemic affect
Green tea	Diabetic cataract	Anti hyperglycemic affect
Adhatoda vasica	Diabetic cataract	Inhibition of AR;Antioxidant activity
Cassia fistula	Diabetic cataract	Inhibition of AR;

Table 4.4 Contd...

Plant	Type of cataract	Mechanism of action
Ocimum sanctum	Diabetic cataract	Decrease in polyol accumilation
Silybum marianum	Diabetic cataract	Antioxidant property
Hydrocotyl bonariensis	Sorbitol induced cataract	Antioxidant property, reduced apoptosis
Curcuma longa	Diabetic cataract	Inhibition of AR; Antioxidant activity
Aralia elata	Diabetic cataract	Inhibition of AR; Antioxidant activity
Brickellia arguta	Diabetic cataract	Inhibition of AR
Emblica officinalis	Diabetic cataract	Inhibition of AR

Cassia fistula was found to show anticataract activity by significantly inhibiting AR activity in rat lens (Gacche *et al.*, 2011). *Ocimum sanctum* and *Silybum marianum* significantly decreased polyol accumulation and increased the GSH levels respectively leading to a protective effect on diabetic cataract (Halder *et al.*, 2003; Huseini *et al.*, 2004). Leaves extract of an AR inhibitor plant *Hydrocotyl bonariensis,* reduced the lens protein precipitation and lens peroxidation and thereby increasing lens antioxidant status and delayed the formation of diabetic cataract. It also led to the reduction in lens apoptosis and epithelial proliferation (Ajani *et al.*, 2009). Treatment of diabetic rats with turmeric or curcumin reversed the diabetic changes with respect to lipid peroxidation, reduced GSH. It also led to the changes in osmotic stress by modification of polyol enzymes and insolublelization of lens proteins was also prevented (Suryanarayana *et al.*, 2005). Tannoid principles from *Emblica officinalis* and flavonoids from *Brickellia arguta* inhibited lens AR activity and thereby inhibited the polyol pathway induced oxidative stress leading to a protective effect on diabetic cataract in rats (Suryanarayana *et al.*, 2007; Rosler *et al.*, 1984). *Aralia elata* extract inhibited lens AR and along with its antioxidant activity and showed a preventive effect on cataractogenesis in xylose containing lens organ cultures and *in vivo* in STZ induced diabetic rats (Chung *et al.*, 2005). Similarly, flavonoids from *Emilia sochifolia* modulated lens opacification by reducing the oxidative stress in selenite-induced cataract (Lija et al., 2006).

Apart from the above-mentioned plants, various phytoconstituents were also found to inhibit AR with a significant protectant role in diabetic cataract (Isai *et al.*, 2009; Yao *et al.*, 2008; Sakthivel *et al.*, 2008; Huang *et al.*, 2007). Quercetin which is a well-known ARI when studied in cataract model, quercetin and its metabolite 3'-O-methyl quercetin inhibited oxidative damage in the lens (Cornish *et al.*, 2002). Other flavonoids such as quercetrin, myricetin and puerariafuran showed the protective effect on diabetic cataract by inhibiting the lens AR (Mohan *et al.,* 1988; Varma *et al.,* 1977; Kim *et al.,* 2010) However puerarin was found to protect against diabetic cataract by exhibiting an anti apoptotic effect on lens epithelial cells (Hao *et al.,* 2011) (Table 4.5).

Table 4.5 Phytochemical with ARI property which studied in diabetic cataract. (dodda *et al.,* 2014).

Compound	Type of cataract	Mechanism of action
Quercetin (1)	Diabetic cataract	Inhibition of oxidative damage; by inhibiting lens AR
Myricetin (2)	Diabetic cataract	Inhibition of lens AR
Quercitrin (23)	Diabetic cataract	Inhibition of lens AR
Rutin (2)	Selenite cataract	Prevention of depletion of GSH, Inhibition of lipid peroxidation.
Fisetin (24)	Radiation cataract	Decreased ROS; modulation of activation of NF-Kb and MAPK
Ellagic acid (13)	Selenite cataract	Inhibition of lipid peroxidation.
Puerarin (25)	Diabetic cataract	Unknown mechanism
Puerariafuran (26)	Diabetic cataract	Inhibition of AR, Inhibition of oxidative damage
Genistein (27)	Diabetic cataract	Increased expression of connexin (Cx) 43

Diabetic Retinopathy

Diabetic retinopathy (DR) is the most common ocular complication in DM and is an important cause of preventable blindness. International classification of Diabetic Retinopathy shown in table 4.6, non proliferative diabetic retinopathy involving intra retinal micro vascular changes and proliferative diabetic retinopathy involving the formation of new vessels or fibrous tissue or both on the retina. DR primarily effects the microvascular circulation of the retina. The factors leading to these changes: thickening of basement membrane of the capillary wall, increased platelet stickiness and changes in RBCs resulting in sluggish microvascular circulation and biochemical changes in the form of activation of polyol pathway resulting in tissue damage. Since the retinal ganglionic cells and endothelial cells are endowed with aldose reductase enzyme, these cells are more prone to damage caused by the activation of polyol pathway leading to DR (Frank 1994; Chew *et al.,* 2010; Funada *et al.,* 1987; Engerman *et al.,* 1993) (Figure 4.3). In table 4.7 summarized advantages and disadvantages of different modalities for diabetic retinopathy screening.

Table 4.6 International classification of Diabetic Retinopathy.
(Anand *et al.*, 2017)

Diabetic Retinopathy	Findings Observable on Dilated Ophthalmoscopy
No apparent DR	No abnormalities
Mild nonproliferative DR	Microaneurysms only
Moderate nonproliferative DR	Microaneurysms and other signs (e.g., dot and blot hemorrhages, hard exudates, cotton wool spots), but less than severe nonproliferative DR
Severe nonproliferative DR	Moderate nonproliferative DR with any of the following: • Intraretinal hemorrhages (≥ 20 in each quadrant); • Definite venous beading (in 2 quadrants); • Intraretinal microvascular abnormalities (in 1 quadrant); • and no signs of proliferative retinopathy
Proliferative DR	Severe nonproliferative DR and 1 or more of the following: • Neovascularization • vitreous/preretinal hemorrhage

Table 4.7 Advantages and disadvantages of different modalities for diabetic retinopathy screening (Squirrell et al., 2003).

Animals models	Characterization of diabetic retinopathy/advantages	Limitations
Retinal photography	1. Effective technique if mydriatic photography is performed with either 35 mm transparencies or digital systems 2. Retinal image can be used in patient education 3. Hard copy can be incorporated into patient record 4. Amenable to audit	High capital set-up costs. Difficulties in reaching all patients who need to be screened. Need to provide regular training for graders. Potential problem retaining motivated personnel for grading.
Optometrist screeners	1. Effective technique if indirect ophthalmoscope/slit lamp biomicroscope used. 2. Accessible, convenient service. 3. Offers holistic package of eye care to the patient.	Requires an elaborate quality control mechanism for the system to be audited.
Combined modalities	1. Effective techniques. 2. Retinal image can be used in patient education. 3. Hard copy can be incorporated into patient record. 4. Amenable to audit. 5. Accessible, convenient service. 6. Offers holistic package of eye care to the patient. 7. Utilizes the well trained, motivated workforce that optometrists represent.	High capital set-up costs. Camera systems might have to rotate around practices, potentially limiting accessibility of the service

Various Mechanism of action of Major Herbal drugs used in Diabetic Retinopathy summarized in table 4.8. Among the various ARIs from natural sources few plants like *Ganoderma lucidum, Tinospora cordifolia, Azardiracta indica, Ganoderma lucidum* were tested for their efficacy in retinopathy in various animal models. However, some plants like *Ocimum sanctum* was found to protect from DR only when given in combination with Vitamin E (Halim et al., 2006). *Tinospora cordifolia* was found to inhibit over expression of angiogenic and inflammatory mediators and thereby prevent retinal oxidative stress exhibiting a protective effect on DR (Agrawal et al., 2012). Similarly, *Ganoderma lucidum* was found to be effective in DR by enhancing the capability of antioxidation in diabetic rats and reducing the damage of retina from oxidation (Yuan et al., 2008).

Table 4.8 Mechanism of action of Major Herbal drugs in Diabetic Retinopathy. (Anand *et al.*, 2017).

S.No.	Plant name	Parts of plant and extract/fraction	Mechanism of action
1.	*Curcuma longa*	Curcumene, Curcumenone, Curcone, Curdione, Cineole, Curzerenone, epiprocurcumenol, eugenol, Camphene, Camphor, Bornel, Procurcumadiol,Procurc umenol, Curcumins, unkonan A, B, & D, B-sitosterol.	antioxidant, possess antiangiogenic properties against SDF-1α.
2.	Trigonella foenum-graecum	4-hydroxyisoleucine	Anti-inflammatory, anti-angiogenic
3.	Ocimum Santum	Eugenol	antioxidant
4.	citrus fruits, apples, onions, parsley, sage, tea, and red wine. Olive oil, grapes, dark cherries, and dark berries such as blueberries, blackberries, and bilberries.	Querecetin	antioxidant, antiapoptotic and anti-inflammatory property
5.	*Camellia sinensis*	epigallocatechin	anti-inflammatory, antioxidative and anticarcinogenic
6.	citrus fruit	Hesperetein	free radical scavenger, antiapoptotic, antioxidant and antiinflammatory

Table 4.8 *Contd...*

S.No.	Plant name	Parts of plant and extract/fraction	Mechanism of action
7.	*Tinospora cordifolia*	(-)Epicatechin, Tinosporin, Isocolumbin, Palmatine,	Antioxidant, Furanolactone, Tinosporin,Tinosporide, Jateorine, Columbin, Clerodane derivatives, Berberine,choline, Tembetarine, Palamtine, Jatrorrhizine
8.	*Panax notoginsen*	ginsenoside Re 14, ginsenoside Rd, ginsenoside Rg1, ginsenoside Rb1 and Notoginsenoside R1	antioxident
9.	*Litsea japonica*	lactones, alkaloids, essential oils, fatty acids, and terpenoids	Antioxidant and antiapoptotic
10.	Astragalus membranaceus, Scrophularia ningpoensis, P. notoginseng and Salvia miltiorrhiza (Fufang Xueshuantong)	P. notoginseng, harpagoside, cryptotanshinone, tanshinone-I, and astragaloside-A .	Anti angiogenesis, anti-oxident
11.	Astragalus membranaceus	Polysaccharides (astragalans I, II and III), saponins (astragalosides I–VIII and isoastragalosides I and II), flavonoids, isoflavonoids, sterols, amino acids, volatile oils and trace elements	Reduce retinal ganglion cell apoptosis Decrease phosphorylation of ERK1/2 Inhibit activation of NF-κB and various cytokines Downregulate the expression of enzyme aldose reductase
12.	Anisodus tanguticus	Anisodamine, anisodine, hyoscyamine, scopolamine, tropine, apoatropine, trichlorophenyl butyryloxytropane and cuscohygrine	Prevent retinal lipid peroxidation Downregulating the expression of plasminogen activator inhibitor-1 (PAI-1) and tissue factor Inhibit the production of TNF-α Activate α7nAChR Downregulate VPO-1

Table 4.8 *Contd...*

S.No.	Plant name	Parts of plant and extract/fraction	Mechanism of action
13.	Ginkgo biloba	Biflavones, terpene trilactones (ginkgolides A, B, C, J, P and Q, and bilobalides), flavonol glycosides (quercetin, catechin) and proanthocyanidins	Downregulate the expression of PAF Reduce the transcriptional expressions of HIF-1α and VEGF
14.	Puerariae lobata	Puerarin, genistein and daidzein	Prevent peroxynitrite-induced cellular apoptosis Attenuate AGE-induced oxidative stress Suppress the activation of NADPH oxidase, VEGF and HIF-1α Inhibit tyrosine kinase Prevent leucocyte–endothelial interaction, vascular dysfunction, leakage and oedema
15.	Salvia miltiorrhiza	Salvianolic acid A, rosmarinic acid	Upregulate endogenous antioxidant enzymes Inhibition of Ang-II-induced NADPH oxidase-4 (Nox4) Preventing endothelial cell proliferation and angiogenesis
16.	Lycium barbarum	Polysaccharides, zeaxanthin, carotene, betaine, cerebroside, beta-sitosterol, pcoumaric, and various vitamins	Upregulation of the expression of anti-apoptotic gene Bcl-2. Downregulate the expression of pro-apoptotic gene Bax Inhibit the activation of cytochrome c/caspase-3-mediated apoptotic pathway.

Phytoconstituents like baicalein, curcumin and hesperetin were effective in DR with baicalein ameliorating inflammatory process and thereby inhibiting vascular abnormality and neuronal loss and in retinal tissues where as curcumin and hesperitin were found to decrease the levels of various mediators like vascular endothelial growth factor (Yang *et al.,* 2009; Kowluru *et al.,* 2007; Kumar *et al.,* 2012). Other substances like quercetin and rosmarinic acid were found to show their effect on DR by prevention of angiogenesis which can be related to the antioxidative properties of the compounds (Chen *et al.,* 2008; Kim *et al.,* 2009; Kern *et al.,* 1999).

Conclusion

As stated earlier, many theories have been proposed and studied to explain mechanisms leading to diabetic complications which includes glucose metabolism through polyol pathway where AR plays a vital role and excessive oxidative stress. While ARIs are the promising targets for the treatment of diabetic complications, most of the developed ARIs show poor or only a partial amelioration and some show unacceptable toxicities. This can be explained by the fact that diverse complications may not share the same and single mechanism. Since it is highly improbable for any single mechanism to explain the pathogenesis associated with diabetic complications, drugs targeted to a specific mechanism often produce unintended effects which is one of the drawbacks for ARIs.

As mentioned in the above reports various plant extracts and their phytoconstituents which showed ARI activity, exhibited their beneficial effect on various complications. However, majority of the ARIs acted by inhibiting oxidative stress or inflammatory changes that occur during DM. As a matter of fact polyol pathway leads to oxidative stress and inhibition of AR leads to the decrease of oxidative stress. But the protective effect of the above mentioned ARIs in diabetic complications is due to the ARI activity thereby decreasing the polyol pathway induced oxidative stress and/or due to the antioxidant property of the compound. Combined with this clinical efficacy of the compounds with either ARI activity or antioxidant property alone seems to be uncertain with various reasons which are beyond the scope of this review. Thus, a molecule with both ARI activity and antioxidative properties could be more effective than a compound with either ARI or antioxidant property alone.

References

Agrawal SS, Naqvi S, Gupta SK, Srivastava S. Prevention and management of diabetic retinopathy in STZ diabetic rats by *Tinospora cordifolia* and its molecular mechanisms. Food Chem Toxicol. 2012;50:3126-32.

Ahmed N. Advanced Glycation end products-role in pathology of diabetic complications. Diabetes Res Clin Pract 2005;67(1):3-21

Ajani EO, Salako AA, Sharlie PD, Akinleye WA, Adeoye AO, Salau BA, *et al.* Chemopreventive and remediation effect of *Hydrocotyl bonariensis* Comm. Ex Lam (Apiaceae) leave extract in galactose-induced cataract. J Ethnopharmacology 2009;123:134-42.

Anand KG, Gupta SK. Diabetic Retinopathy: Role of Traditional Medicinal Plants in its management and their molecular mechanism. *International Journal of Pharmaceutical Science Invention.* 2017; 6(6): 01-14.

Anjaneyulu M, Chopra K. Quercetin, a bioflavonoid, attenuates thermal hyperalgesia in a mouse model of diabetic neuropathic pain. Prog Neuropsychopharmacol Biol Psychiatry 2003;27(6):1001-5.

Anjaneyulu M, Chopra K. Quercetin, an anti-oxidant bioflavonoid, attenuates diabetic nephropathy in rats. Clin Exp Pharmacol Physiol 2004;31(4):244-8.

Bagdas D, Cinkilic N, Ozboluk HY, Ozyigit MO, Gurun MS. Antihyperalgesic activity of chlorogenic acid in experimental neuropathic pain. J Nat Med 2012; doi: 10.1007/s11418-012-0726-z.

Boel E, Selmer J, Flodgaard HJ, Jensen T. Diabetic late complications: will aldose reductase inhibitors or inhibitors of advanced glycosylation endproduct formation hold promise? J Diabetes Complications 1995;9(2):104-29.

Brownlee M. Biochemistry and molecular cell biology of diabetic complications. Nature 2001;414:813-20.

Celia G, Cummings E, David AP, Jaipaul S. Beneficial effect and mechanism of action of *Momordica charantia* in the treatment of diabetes mellitus: a mini review. Int J Diabetes & Metabolism 2003;11:46-55.

Chao CY, Mong MC, Chan KC, Yin MC. Anti-glycative and anti-inflammatory effects of caffeic acid and ellagic acid in kidney of diabetic mice. Mol Nutr Food Res 2010;54(3):388-95.

Chen L, Lan Z, Zhou Y, Li F, Zhang X, Zhang C, *et al.* Astilbin attenuates hyperuricemia and ameliorates nephropathy in fructose-induced hyperuricemic rats. Planta Med 2011;77(16):1769-73.

Chen Y, Li XX, Xing NZ, Cao XG. Quercetin inhibits choroidal and retinal angiogenesis *in vitro.* Graefes Arch Clin Exp Ophthalmol 2008;246(3):373-8.

Chethan S, Dharmesh SM, Malleshi NG. Inhibition of aldose reductase from cataracted eye lenses by finger millet (*Eleusine coracana*) polyphenols. Bioorg Med Chem 2008;16(23):10085-90.

Chew EY, Ambrosius WT, Davis MD, Danis RP, Gangaputra S, Greven CM, Hubbard L, Esser BA, Lovato JF, Perdue LH, Goff DC Jr, Cushman WC, Ginsberg HN, Elam MB, Genuth S, Gerstein HC, Schubart U, Fine LJ. Effects of medical therapies on retinopathy progression in type 2 diabetes. N Eng J Med 2010; 363: 233-44.

Chiu J, Khan ZA, Farhangkhoee H, Chakrabarti S. Curcumin prevents diabetes-associated abnormalities in the kidneys by inhibiting p300 and nuclear factor-kappaB. Nutrition 2009;25(9):964-72.

Choi R, Kim BH, Naowaboot J, Lee MY, Hyun MR, Cho EJ, *et al.* Effects of ferulic acid on diabetic nephropathy in a rat model of type 2 diabetes. Exp Mol Med 2011;43(12):676-83.

Chung YS, Choi YH, Lee SJ, Choi SA, Lee JH, Kim H, *et al.* Water extract of *Aralia elata* prevents cataractogenesis *in vitro* and *in vivo.* J Ethnopharmacology 2005;101:49-54.

Cornish KM, Williamson G, Sanderson J. Quercetin metabolism in the lens: role in inhibition of hydrogen peroxide induced cataract. Free Radic Biol Med 2002;33(1):63-70.

Dodda D, Ciddi V. Plants Used in the Management of Diabetic Complications. Indian   Journal of Pharmaceutical Sciences 2014; 76(2):97-106.

Du ZY, Bao YD, Liu Z, Qiao W, Ma L, Huang ZS, *et al.* Curcumin analogs as potent aldose reductase inhibitors. Arch Pharm (Weinheim) 2006;339(3):123-8.

Ederer F, Hiller R, Taylor HR. Senile lens changes and diabetes in two population studies. Am J Ophthalmol 1981;91:381-95.

Edwards JL, Vincent AM, Cheng HT, Feldman EL. Diabetic neuropathy: mechanisms to management. Pharmacol Ther 2008;120(1):1-34.

Engerman RL, Kern TS. Aldose reductase inhibition fails to prevent retinopathy in diabetic and galactosemic dogs. Diabetes 1993;42:820-5.

Frank RN. Etiologic mechanisms in diabetic retinopathy. In: Ryan SJ, editor. Retina, 2nd ed. St. Louis, CV Mosby; 1994. 1243-76.

Funada M, Okamoto I, Fujinaga Y, Yamana T. Effects of aldose reductase inhibitor (M79175) on ERG oscillatory potential abnormalities in streptozotocin fructose- induced diabetes in rats. lpn J Ophthalmol 1987;31:305- 14.

Gabbay KH. The sorbitol pathway and the complications of diabetes. N Engl J Med 1973;288(16):831-6.

Gacche RN, Dhole NA. Aldose reductase inhibitory, anticataract and antioxidant potential of selected medicinal plants from the Marathwada region, India. Nat Prod Res 2011;25:760-3.

Garcia SF, Virág L, Jagtap P, Szabó E, Mabley JG, Liaudet L, *et al.* Diabetic endothelial dysfunction: the role of poly(ADP-ribose) polymerase activation. Nat Med 2001; 7(1):108-13.

Goodarzi MT, Zal F, Malakooti M, Safari MR, Sadeghian S. Inhibitory activity of flavonoids on the lens aldose reductase of healthy and diabetic rats. Acta Medica Iranica 2006;44(1):41-5.

Halder N, Joshi S, Gupta SK. Lens aldose reductase inhibiting potential of some indigenous plants. J Ethnopharmacol 2003; 86:113-6.

Halim EM, Mukhopadhyay AK. Effect of *Ocimum sanctum* (Tulsi) and Vitamin E on biochemical parameters and retinopathy in streptozotocin induced diabetic rats. Indian J Clin Biochem 2006;21(2):181-8.

Hao LN, He SZ, Shen YH, Zhang YQ, Wang ZY, Wang YH. Protective effects of puerarin on lens epithelial cells in rat diabetic cataract. Zhonghua Yan Ke Za Zhi 2011;47(4):320-6.

Haraguchi H, Ohmi I, Fukuda A, Tamura Y, Mizutani K, Tanaka O, *et al.* Inhibition of aldose reductase and sorbitol accumulation by astilbin and taxifolin dihydroflavonols in *Engelhardtia chrysolepis*. Biosci Biotechnol Biochem 1997;61(4):651-4.

Haraguchi H, Ohmi I, Sakai S, Fukuda A, Toihara Y, Fujimoto T, *et al.* Effect of *Polygonum hydropiper* sulfated flavonoids on lens aldose reductase and related enzymes. J Nat Prod 1996;59(4):443-5.

Hase M, Babazono T, Karibe S, Kinae N, Iwamoto Y. Renoprotective effects of tea catechin in streptozotocin- induced diabetic rats. Int Urol Nephrol 2006;38:693-9.

Huang R, Shi F, Lei T, Song Y, Hughes CL, Liu G. Effect of the isoflavone genistein against galactose-induced cataracts in rats. Exp Biol Med 2007;232(1):118-25.

Huseini HF, Zaree AB, Zarch AB, Heshmat R. The effect of herbal medicine *Silybum marianum* (L.) Gaertn. seed extract on galactose induced cataract formation in rat. J Med Plants 2004; 3: 58-62.

Intensive blood-glucose control with sulphonylureas or insulin compared with conventional treatment and risk of complications in patients with type 2 diabetes (UKPDS 33). UK Prospective Diabetes Study (UKPDS) Group. Lancet 1998;352: 837-53.

Isai M, Sakthivel M, Ramesh E, Thomas PA, Geraldine P. Prevention of selenite-induced cataractogenesis by rutin in Wistar rats. Molecular Vision 2009;15:2570-7.

Je HD, Shin CY, Park SY, Yim SH, Kum C, Huh IH, *et al.* Combination of vitamin C and rutin on neuropathy and lung damage of diabetes mellitus rats. Arch Pharm Res 2002;25(2):184-90.

Joe A, Vinson, Juan Zhang. Black and Green Teas Equally Inhibit Diabetic Cataracts in a Streptozotocin-Induced Rat Model of Diabetes. J Agric Food Chem 2005;53:3710-3.

Jung 2002;Asaba K, Tojo A, Onozato ML, Goto A, Quinn MT, Fujita T, *et al.* Effects of NADPH oxidase inhibitor in diabetic nephropathy. Kidney Int 2005;67(5):1890-8.Jung SH, Lee YS, Lee S, Lim SS, Kim YS, Shin KH. Isoflavonoids from the rhizomes of *Belamcanda chinensis* and their effects on aldose reductase and sorbitol accumulation in streptozotocin induced diabetic rat tissues. Arch Pharm Res 2002;25(3):306-12.Kaeidi A, Esmaeili-Mahani S, Sheibani V, Abbasnejad M, Rasoulian B, Hajializadeh Z, *et al.* Olive (*Olea europaea* L.) leaf extract attenuates early diabetic neuropathic pain through prevention of high glucose-induced apoptosis: *in vitro* and *in vivo* studies. J Ethnopharmacol 2011;136(1):188-96.

Kandhare AD, Raygude KS, Ghosh P, Ghule AE, Bodhankar SL. Neuroprotective effect of naringin by modulation of endogenous biomarkers in streptozotocin induced painful diabetic neuropathy. Fitoterapia 2012;83(4):650-9.

Kang DG, Lee AS, Mun YJ, Woo WH, Kim YC, Sohn EJ, *et al.* Butein ameliorates renal concentrating ability in cisplatin-induced acute renal failure in rats. Biol Pharm Bull 2004;27(3):366-70.

Kapor-Drezgic J, Zhou X, Babazono T, Dlugosz JA, Hohman T, Whiteside C. Effect of high glucose on mesangial cell protein kinase C-delta and -epsilon is polyol pathway-dependent. J Am Soc Nephrol 1999;10:1193-203.

Kasajima H, Yamagisi S, Sugai S, Yagihashi N, Yagihashi S. Enhanced in situ expression of aldose reductase in peripheral nerve and renal glomeruli in diabetic patients. Virchows Arch 2001;439:46-54.

Kato A, Higuchi Y, Gato H, Kizu H, Okamoto T, Asano N, *et al.* Inhibitory effects of *Zingiber officinale* Roscoe derived components on aldose reductase activity *in vitro* and *in vivo*. J Agric Food Chem 2006;54: 6640-4.

Kern TS, Engerman RL. Aldose reductase and the development of renal disease in diabetic dogs. J Diabetes Complications 1999;13(1):10-6.

Kim JH, Lee BJ, Kim JH, Yu YS, Kim MY, Kim KW. Rosmarinic acid suppresses retinal neovascularization via cell cycle arrest with increase of p21 (WAF1) expression. Eur J Pharmacol 2009;615:150-4.

Kim NH, Kim YS, Lee YM, Jang DS, Kim JS. Inhibition of aldose reductase and xylose-induced lens opacity by puerariafuran from the roots of *Pueraria lobata*. Biol Pharm Bull 2010;33(9):1605-9.

Koukoulitsa C, Zika C, Geromichalos GD, Demopoulos VJ, Skaltsa H. Evaluation of aldose reductase inhibition and docking studies of some secondary metabolites, isolated from *Origanum vulgare* L. ssp. hirtum. Bioorg Med Chem 2006;14(5):1653-9.

Kowluru RA, Kanwar M. Effects of curcumin on retinal oxidative stress and inflammation in diabetes. Nutr Metab 2007;4:8.

Krolewski AS, Warram JH, Christlieb AR, Busick EJ, Kahn CR The changing natural history of nephropathy in type I diabetes. Am J Med 1985;78:785-94.

Lee AY, Chung SS. Contributions of polyol pathway to oxidative stress in diabetic cataract. Faseb J 1999;13:23-30.

Lee EH, Song DG, Lee JY, Pan CH, Um BH, Jung SH. Inhibitory effect of the compounds isolated from *Rhus verniciflua* on aldose reductase and advanced glycation endproducts. Biol Pharm Bull 2008;31(8):1626-30.

Lee HS. Rat lens aldose reductase inhibitory activities of *Coptis japonica* root-derived isoquiniline alkaloids. J Agric Food Chem 2002;50:7013-6.

Li R, Yuan C, Dong C, Shuang S, Choi MM. *In vivo* antioxidative effect of isoquercitrin on cadmium-induced oxidative damage to mouse liver and kidney. Naunyn Schmiedebergs Arch Pharmacol 2011;383(5):437-45.

Li X, Cui X, Sun X, Li X, Zhu Q, Li W. Mangiferin prevents diabetic nephropathy progression in streptozotocin-induced diabetic rats. Phytother Res 2010;24(6):893-9.

Lija Y, Biju PG, Reeni A, Cibin TR, Sahasranamam V, Abraham A. Modulation of selenite cataract by the flavonoid fraction of *Emilia sonchifolia* in experimental animal models. Phytother Res 2006;20(12):1091-5.

Logendra S, Ribnicky DM, Yang H, Poulev A, Ma J, Kennelly EJ, *et al.* Bioassay-guided isolation of aldose reductase inhibitors from *Artemisia dracunculus.* Phytochemistry 2006;67(14):1539-46.

Majid T, Hasan A, Alireza K, Ahmad T. Rosmarinic Acid Ameliorates Diabetic Nephropathy in Uninephrectomized Diabetic Rats. Iran J Basic Med Sci 2011;14(3):275-83.

Mohan M, Gupta SK, Agnihotri S, Joshi S, Uppal RK. Anticataract action of topical quercetin and myricetin in galactosemic rats. Med Sci Res 1988;6:685-6.

Morikawa T, Kishi A, Pongpiriyadacha Y, Matsuda H, Yoshikawa M. Structures of new friedelane-type triterpenes and eudesmane-type sesquiterpene and aldose reductase inhibitors from *Salacia chinensis.* J Nat Prod 2003;66(9):1191-6.

Murata M, Iries J, Homma S. Aldose reductase inhibitors from green tea. J Food Sci Technol 1994;27:401-5.

Nangle MR, Gibson TM, Cotter MA, Cameron NE. Effects of eugenol on nerve and vascular dysfunction in streptozotocin-diabetic rats. Planta Med 2006;72(6):494-500.

Nanjundan PK, Arunachalam A, Thakur RS. Antinociceptive Property of *Trigonella foenum graecum* (Fenugreek seeds) in High Fat Diet-Fed/Low Dose Streptozotocin Induced Diabetic Neuropathy in Rats. Pharmacologyonline 2009;2:24-36.

Nathan DM, Genuth S, Lachin J, Cleary P, Crofford O, Davis M, Rand L, Siebert C. The Diabetes Control and Complications Trial Research Group. The effect of intensive treatment of diabetes on the development and progression of long-term complications in insulin-dependent diabetes mellitus. N Engl J Med 1993;329:977-86.

Oates PJ, Mylari BL. Aldose reductase inhibitors: therapeutic implications for diabetic complications. Expert Opin Investig Drugs 1999;8:2095-119.

Oka M, Kato N. Aldose reductase inhibitors. J Enzyme Inhib 2001;16(6):465-73.

Ozcan F, Ozmen A, Akkaya B, Aliciguzel Y, Aslan M. Beneficial effect of myricetin on renal functions in streptozotocin-induced diabetes. Clin Exp Med 2012;12(4):265-72.

Piyush P, Nurudin J, Shailesh M, Tushar G, Yagnik B. Cataract: A major secondary diabetic complication. International Current Pharmaceutical Journal. 2012; 1(7): 180-185.

Pontiroli AE, Calderara A, Pozza G. Secondary failure of oral hypoglycaemic agents: frequency, possible causes, and management. Diabetes Metab Rev 1994;10(1):31-43.

Qattan KA, Thomson M, Muslim A.Garlic (*Allium sativum*) and ginger (*Zingiber officinale*) attenuate structural nephropathy progression in streptozotocin-induced diabetic rats. e-SPEN, the European e-J Clin Nutr Metabol 2008;3:e62-e71.

Rosenstock PJ. Aldose reductase inhibitors and diabetic complications. Am J Med 1987;83:298-306.

Rosler KH, Goodwin RS, Mabry TJ, Varma SD, Norris J. Flavonoids with anti-cataract activity from *Brickellia arguta*. J Nat Prod 1984;47(2):316-9.

Saber AS, Hawazen AL. Protective Effect of Rosemary (*Rosmarinus Officinalis*) Leaves Extract on Carbon Tetrachloride - Induced Nephrotoxicity in Albino Rats. Life Science Journal 2012;9(1):779-85.

Sakthivel M, Elanchezhian R, Ramesh E, Isai M, Jesudasan CN, Thomas PA, Geraldine P. Prevention of selenite-induced cataractogenesis in Wistar rats by the polyphenol, ellagic acid. Exp Eye Res. 2008;86(2):251-9

Saraswat M, Muthenna P, Suryanarayana P, Petrash JM, Reddy GB. Dietary sources of aldose reductase inhibitors: prospects for alleviating diabetic complications. Asia Pac J Clin Nutr 2008;17:558-65.

Shahidul Islam Md. Animal Models of Diabetic Neuropathy: Progress Since 1960s. Journal of Diabetes Research. 2013; Article ID 149452, 9 pages.

Sharma AK, Bharti S, Ojha S, Bhatia J, Kumar N, Ray R, *et al*. Up-regulation of PPARγ, heat shock protein-27 and -72 by naringin attenuates insulin resistance, β-cell dysfunction, hepatic steatosis and kidney damage in a rat model of type 2 diabetes Br J Nutr. 2011;106(11):1713-23.

Sharma S, Kulkarni SK, Agrewala JN, Chopra K. Curcumin attenuates thermal hyperalgesia in a diabetic mouse model of neuropathic pain. Eur J Pharmacol 2006;536(3):256-61.

Shaw JE, Sicree RA, Zimmet PZ. Global estimates of the prevalence of diabetes for 2010 and 2030. Diabetes research and clinical practice 2010;87:4–14.

Squirrell DM, Talbot JF. Screening for diabetic retinopathy. Journal of the Royal Society of Medicine 2003; 96(6): 273–276.

Stavniichuk R, Drel VR, Shevalye H, Maksimchyk Y, Kuchmerovska TM, Nadler JL, *et al*. Baicalein alleviates diabetic peripheral neuropathy through inhibition of oxidative-nitrosative stress and p38 MAPK activation. Exp Neurol 2011; 230(1):106-13.

Suresh Babu P, Srinivasan K. Amelioration of renal lesions associated with diabetes by dietary curcumin in streptozotocin diabetic rats. Mol Cell Biochem 1998;181:87-96.

Suryanarayana P, Saraswat M, Mrudula T, Krishna TP, Krishnaswamy K, Reddy GB. Curcumin and turmeric delay streptozotocin-induced diabetic cataract in rats. Invest Ophthalmol Vis Sci 2005;46(6):2092-9.

Suryanarayana P, Saraswat M, Petrash JM, Reddy GB. *Emblica officinalis* and its enriched tannoids delay streptozotocin-induced diabetic cataract in rats. Mol Vis 2007;13:1291-7.

Tomás-Barberán FA, López-Gómez C, Villar A, Tomás-Lorente F. Inhibition of lens aldose reductase by Labiatae flavonoids. Planta Med 1986;(3):239-40.

Tourandokht B, and Mehrdad R. Chronic Oral Epigallocatechin-gallate alleviates streptozotocin-induced diabetic neuropathic hyperalgesia in rat: Involvement of oxidative stress. Iranian Journal of Pharmaceutical Research 2012;11(4):1243-53.

Ueda H, Kuroiwa E, Tachibana Y, Kawanishi K, Ayala F, Moriyasu M. Aldose reductase inhibitors from the leaves of *Myrciaria dubia* (H. B. & K.) McVaugh. Phytomedicine 2004;11:652-6.

Uzar E, Alp H, Cevik MU, Fırat U, Evliyaoglu O, Tufek A, *et al*. Ellagic acid attenuates oxidative stress on brain and sciatic nerve and improves histopathology of brain in streptozotocin-induced diabetic rats. Neurol Sci 2012;33(3):567-74.

Varma SD, Mikuni I, Kinoshita JH. Flavonoids as inhibitors of lens aldose reductase. Science 1975;188:1215-16.

Varma SD, Mizuno A, Kinoshita JH. Diabetic Cataracts and Flavonoids. Science 1977;195:205-6.

Wang GG, Lu XH, Li W, Zhao X, Zhang C. Protective Effects of Luteolin on Diabetic Nephropathy in STZ-Induced Diabetic Rats. Evid Based Complement Alternat Med 2011; 323171. doi: 10.1155/2011/323171.

Watcho P, Stavniichuk R, Tane P, Shevalye H, Maksimchyk Y, Pacher P, *et al*. IG. Evaluation of PMI-5011, an ethanolic extract of *Artemisia dracunculus* L., on peripheral neuropathy in streptozotocin-diabetic mice. Int J Mol Med 2011;27(3):299-307.

Wilson DK, Bohren KM, Gabbay KH, Quiocho FA. An unlikely sugar substrate site in the 1.65 A structure of the human aldose reductase holo enzyme implicated in diabetic complications. Science 1992; 257: 81-4.

Wu D, Wen W, Qi CL, Zhao RX, Lü JH, Zhong CY, *et al*. Ameliorative effect of berberine on renal damage in rats with diabetes induced by high-fat diet and streptozotocin. Phytomedicine 2012;19:712-8.

Xie Y, Jingdan S, Wenpu C, AFRC. Effects of Puerarin injection on diabetic peripheral neuropathy:Analysis of 31 cases. Journal of Guangdong Medical College 1998 -Z1.

Yamabe N, Yokozawa T, Oya T, Kim M. Therapeutic potential of (-)-epigallocatechin 3-O-gallate on renal damage in diabetic nephropathy model rats. J Pharmacol Exp Ther 2006;319(1):228-36.

Yang 2009;Kowluru 2007;Kumar B, Gupta SK, Srinivasan BP, Nag TC, Srivastava S, Saxena R. Hesperetin ameliorates hyperglycemia induced retinal vasculopathy via anti-angiogenic effects in experimental diabetic rats. Vascul Pharmacol 2012;57:201-7.

Yang LP, Sun HL, Wu LM, Guo XJ, Dou HL, Tso MO, *et al*. Baicalein reduces inflammatory process in a rodent model of diabetic retinopathy. Invest Ophthalmol Vis Sci 2009;50(5):2319-27.

Yanhu D, Linan P, Xiujun W. Primary observation of therapeutic effect of baicalin on diabetic peripheral neuropathy. Chinese J of Diabetes 1999; 06.

Yao K, Zhang L, Zhang Y, Ye P, Zhu N. The flavonoid fisetin inhibits UV radiation-induced oxidative stress and the activation of NF-kappaB and MAPK signaling in human lens epithelial cells. Mol Vis.2008;14:1865-71.

Yoshikawa M, Morikawa T, Murakami T, Toguchida I, Harima S, Matsuda H. Medicinal flowers. I. Aldose reductase inhibitors and three new eudesmane-type sesquiterpenes, kikkanols A, B, and C, from the flowers of *Chrysanthemum indicum* L. Chem Pharm Bull 1999;47(3):340-5.

Yuan YX, Wang SQ. Effects of *Ganoderma lucidum* Spores on Antioxidatizing Reaction in the Retinal Tissue of Diabetic Rats. Chin Arch Trad Chin Med 2008;26(3):637-8.

Chapter 5

Herbal Medicine in Diabetic Foot Complications

5.1 Introduction

Diabetic Foot Ulcer (DFU) is one of the most common and devastating complications of Diabetes Mellitus (DM), which has indicated an increasing trend in the past decades (Rice *et al.*, 2014). Recent reports have shown that more than 15% of patients with DM had DFU during their lifetime (Leone *et al.*, 2012). Although the exact figures are difficult to obtain for the prevalence of DFU, its prevalence has been reported as 4% to 27% in different parts of the world (Shahi *et al.*, 2012; Richard *et al.*, 2008; Nather *et al.*, 2008; Bakri *et al.*, 2012). DFU mainly caused by ischemic, neuropathic or combined neuroischemic abnormalities (Schaper *et al.*, 2003). The healing of ulcer in patients with diabetes is reported to be poor (Greer *et al.*, 2013). It is reported that a considerable number of patients with DFU remain unhealed after 12 weeks of treatment, and in treatable cases healing occurs in 2 or 5 months virtually (Moura *et al.*, 2013). Based on one study conducted in the USA, standard care heals only between 24% and 31% of DFU (Baquerizo *et al.*, 2014). Ultimately, unhealed DFU in the most cases lead to infection, gangrene, amputation, and even death if the necessary care is not provided (Snyder *et al.*, 2009). The risk of lower extremity amputation reports 15 to 46 times higher in patients with diabetes than in persons without diabetes (Leone *et al.*, 2012). Furthermore, non-healing ulcers affect patient quality of life and productivity and represent a substantial financial burden on the health care system (Driver *et al.*, 2010; Siersma *et al.*, 2014). So, healing of ulcer in patients with diabetes can prevent the most serious complications of this problem. The primary management goals for DFU are to obtain wound closure as expeditiously as possible (Alavi *et al.*, 2014). As diabetes is a multi-organ systemic disease, all comorbidities that affect wound healing must be managed by a multi-disciplinary team for optimal outcomes with DFU. Based on National Institute for Health and Clinical Excellence (NICE) strategies, the management of DFU should be done immediately with a multidisciplinary team that consists of a general practitioner, a nurse, an educator, an orthotic specialist, a podiatrist, and consultations with other specialists such as vascular surgeons, infectious disease specialists, dermatologists, endocrinologists, dieticians, and orthopedic specialists. Multi-disciplinary approaches for management of DFU include control of patient's blood glucose, antibiotics therapy, off-loading devices, wound debridement, advanced dressings as well as surgery in selected cases (Sumpio *et al.*, 2004; Wraight *et al.*, 2005). Furthermore, many adjunctive therapies could be used for rapid healing of DFU including hyperbaric oxygen therapy (HBOT) (O'Reilly *et al.*, 2013), Negative Pressure Wound Therapy (NPWT) (Zhang *et al.*, 2014), recombinant Human Platelet-Derived Growth Factor-BB (rPDGF-BB) [Kirsner 2010], Electrical Stimulation (ES) (Barnes *et al.*, 2014) and Bio-Engineered Skin (BES) (Widgerow 2014). In spite of these various options for healing of DFU, studies showed the poor healing of DFU (Moura *et al.*, 2013; Baquerizo *et al.*, 2014). Besides, the rising costs of these approaches impose a lot of costs to patients and health care systems, and urge the need of new therapeutic agents (Driver *et al.*, 2010). Therefore, design of low cost and effective methods to heal DFU seems to be essential that is only possible with natural therapy. To date, various herbal products have been used in the management and treatment of DFU and following section describe about herbal medicine used in diabetic foot complication.

Herbal Medicine in Diabetic Foot Complications

This study was carried out at multi-centric randomized controlled trial in Iran and UAE. To evaluate the efficacy of intravenous Semelil (ANGIPARSTM), a naive herbal extract to accelerate healing of diabetic foot ulcers. Sixteen diabetic patients were treated with intravenous Semelil, and nine other patients were treated with placebo as control group. Both groups were treated by wound debridement and irrigation with normal saline solution, systemic antibiotic therapy and daily wound dressing. Before and after intervention, the foot ulcer surface area was measured, by digital photography, mapping and planimetry. After 4 weeks, the mean foot ulcer surface area decreased from 479.93±379.75 mm to 198.93±143.75 mm, in the intervention group (p = 0.000) and from 766.22±960.50 mm to 689.11±846.74 mm, in the control group (p = 0.076). Average wound closure in the treatment group was significantly greater than placebo group. This herbal extract by intravenous rout in combination with conventional therapy is more effective than conventional therapy by itself probably without side effect (Larijani *et al.*, 2008).

The herbs Radix Astragali (RA) and Radix Rehmanniae (RR) have long been used in traditional Chinese Medicine and serve as the principal herbs in treating diabetic foot ulcer. A simplified 2-herb formula (NF3) comprising of RA and RR in the ratio of 2:1 was used for this study. NF3 was examined for a chemically induced diabetic foot ulcer rat model. *In vivo* results demonstrated a significant reduction of wound area at day 8 in NF3 (0.98 g/kg) group as compared to control (p < 0.01) (Jacqueline *et al.,* 2011). In another study, Kit-Man *et al.,* 2012 reported that, the possible synergistic effect between AR and RR in NF3 to promote diabetic wound healing and to identify the principal herb in the formula by evaluating the potencies of individual AR and RR in different mechanistic studies. A chemically induced diabetic foot ulcer rat model was used to examine the wound healing effect of NF3 and its individual herbs AR and RR. In the foot ulcer animal model, neither AR nor RR at clinical relevant dose (0.98 g/kg) promoted diabetic wound healing. However, when they were used in combination as NF3, synergistic interaction was demonstrated, of which NF3 could significantly reduce the wound area of rats when compared to water group (p < 0.01).

The study was carried out on 50 adult patients who had grade I diabetic foot ulcers in Egypt. The sample was divided equally into two groups, study and control groups. The study group was treated by ozonated olive oil ointment, and control group was treated by hospital routine solutions (saline 0.9%, betadine 10%) once in a day. This study revealed that, although the two dressing techniques (ozonated olive oil ointment and betadine 10% wet dressing techniques) were effective on the healing process of grade I diabetic foot ulcers, yet ozonated olive oil solution had better healing effect than conventional solution (Aziza *et al.,* 2011).

Tangzu Yuyang Ointment (TYO) is a topical Chinese herbal medicine (CHM) compound made from nine herbal medicines and two natural minerals. Ingredients of TYO formula and their phytochemical constituents and pharmacological action summarized in table 5.1. Clinical trial was conducted at seven centers in the China mainland. Fifty-seven patients with chronic diabetic foot ulcers of Wagner's ulcer grade 1–3 were enrolled in this study. Patients who were randomly assigned to the control group (n = 28) received standard wound therapy (SWT), whereas those randomized to the treatment group (n = 28) received SWT plus topical TYO. Only 48 patients who finished 24 weeks of observations were entered for data analysis. The TYO and SWT groups were comparable for baseline characteristics. Ulcer improvement was 79.2% in the TYO group and 41.7% in the SWT group (P = 0.017) at 12 weeks, and 91.7% vs. 62.5% (P = 0.036) at 24 weeks. The number of ulcers that were completely healed at 4, 12 and 24 weeks was similar in both groups, as were the numbers of adverse events. Healing time was 96±56 days (n = 19) in the TYO group and 75±53 days (n = 14) in the SWT group (P = 0.271). TYO plus SWT is more effective than SWT in the management of chronic diabetic foot ulcers and has few side-effects. (Shufa *et al.,* 2011).

Table 5.1 Ingredients of TYO formula and their phytochemical constituents and pharmacological action. (Shufa *et al.*, 2011).

Chinese names	Scientific names	part used	Ratio	Phytochemical constituents	Pharmacological action in wound healing
Huanglian	Coptis chinensis Franch.	root	30	Berberine, coptisine, worrenine, palmatine, ferulic acid, mognoflorine	Sterilization, anti inflammaton, analgesia, nourish nerve, inhibition of platelet aggregation
Chuanxiong	Ligusticum chuanxiong Hort.	Root	30	Tetramethyl pyrazine, Leucylphenyl alanine anhyolride, perlolyrine, ferulic acid.	Inhibition of platelet aggregation, antithrombosis, inhibition of bacteria
Cangzhu	Atractylodes lancea (Thund.) DC.	root	50	Atractylol,β-eudesmol, hinesol, atractylodon, atractylodin	Sterilization, antioxidant, modify cellular glucose homeostasis
Sanqi	Panax notoginseng (Burk.) F.H. Chen	root	20	Ginsenoside, sanehinam A, daueosterol	Hemostatic mechanism, anticoagulant, anti inflammation, antioxidant, anti-immune.
Danggui	Angelica sinensis (Oliv.) Diels	root	20	Ferulic acid, succininc, nicotinic acid, butylidenephthalide, folinic acid	Inhibition of platelet aggregation, antithrombosis, analgesia, inhibition of bacteria, antioxidant
Zicao	Arnebia euchroma (Royle) Johnst	root	10	Skikonin, acetylshikonin, βhydroxyisovalerylshikonin,teracrylshikenin	Anti-inflammation, inhibition of bacteria.
Huangbo	Phellodendron chinense Schneid	bark	20	Berberine, magnoflorine, palmatine,phellodendrine, obaculactone,obacunone	Inhibition of bacteria, anti-immune, anti-inflammation.

Table 5.1 Contd...

Chinese names	Scientific names	part used	Ratio	Phytochemical constituents	Pharmacological action in wound healing
Dahuang	Rheum officinale Baill.	root	15	Rhein, emodin, chrysophanol, chrysaron, aloe-emodin, physcion.	Hemostatic mechanism, anticoagulant, inhibition of bacteria, antiinflammation, antioxidant.
Bingpian	Borneolum syntheticum		2	d-Borneol, l-borneol.	Inhibition of bacteria, antiinflammation, analgesia, promote nerve cell growth, increase penetration of agent through skin.
Xuejie	Daemonorops draco Bl.	resin	30	Dracorubin, dracorhodin, nordracorubin, nordracorhodin.	Hemostatic mechanism, anticoagulant, inhibition of bacteria, antiinflammation, analgesia.
Duanshigao	*Gypsum fibrosum praeparatum*		**150**	**Calcium sulfate**	**Adsorption effusion, hemostatic mechanism.**

Double-blind randomized clinical trial study was conducted in Diabetes Clinic of Ahvaz Golestan hospital, Iran, in 2014. Thirty-four patients with DFU of Wagner's ulcer grade 1 or 2 were enrolled in study. Patients who were randomly assigned to intervention group (n = 17) received topical olive oil in addition to routine cares, whereas patients in control group (n = 17) just received routine cares. Intervention was done once a day for 4 weeks in both groups, and in the end of each week; the ulcers were assessed and scored. Data was collected by demographic and clinical characteristics checklists as well as diabetic foot ulcer healing checklist, and was analyzed by SPSS version 19 software using descriptive (mean and standard deviation) and analytic (student's sample t-test, chi-square and repeated-measures analysis of variance) statistics. At the end of 4th week, there was a significant differences between two groups regarding to 3 parameters of ulcer including degree (P = 0.03), color (P = 0.04) and surrounding tissues (P < 0.001) as well as total status of ulcer (P = 0.001), while related to ulcer drainages no significant difference was seen between the two groups (P = 0.072). At the end of the follow up, olive oil significantly decreased ulcer area (P = 0.01) and depth (P = 0.02) compared with control group. Complete ulcer healing in the intervention group was significantly greater than control group (73.3% vs. 13.3%, P = 0.003) at the end of follow up shown in figure 5.1. Also, there were no adverse effects to report during the study in intervention group (Morteza *et al.*, 2015).

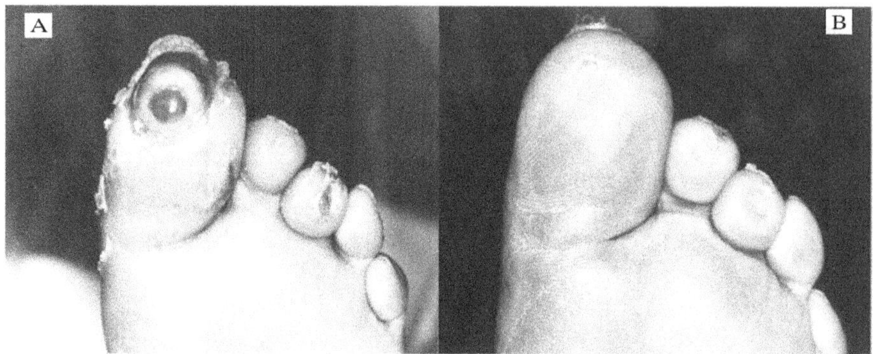

Figure 5.1 Complete healing in a patient treated with topical olive oil before intervention (A) and at the end of follow up (B). (Morteza *et al.*, 2015).

References

Alavi A, Sibbald RG, Mayer D, Goodman L, Botros M, Armstrong DG. Diabetic foot ulcers: Part II. Management. J Am Acad Dermatol. 2014; 70(21):e1–24.

Aziza ES, Nahad E, Nabila AB, Wael Sh. Comparative Study of Ozonated Olive Oil Ointment versus Conventional Dressing Methods on the Healing of Grade I Diabetic Foot Ulcers. Researcher, 2011; 3(8): 16-30.

Bakri FG, Allan AH, Khader YS, Younes NA, Ajlouni KM. Prevalence of Diabetic Foot Ulcer and its Associated Risk Factors among Diabetic Patients in Jordan. J Med J. 2012; 46: 118–125.

Baquerizo Nole KL, Kirsner RS. Advanced wound care therapies in non-healing lower extremity ulcers: high expectations, low evidence. Evid Based Med. 2014; 19: 91.

Barnes R, Shahin Y, Gohil R, Chetter I. Electrical stimulation vs. standard care for chronic ulcer healing: a systematic review and meta-analysis of randomised controlled trials. Eur J Clin Invest. 2014; 44: 429–440.

Driver VR, Fabbi M, Lavery LA, Gibbons G. The costs of diabetic foot: the economic case for the limb salvages team. J Vasc Surg. 2010; 52(3): 17–22.

Greer N, Foman NA, MacDonald R, Dorrian J, Fitzgerald P, Rutks I. Advanced wound care therapies for nonhealing diabetic, venous, and arterial ulcers: a systematic review. Ann Intern Med. 2013; 159: 532–542.

Jacqueline Chor Wing Tam, Kit Man Laua, Cheuk Lun Liu, Ming Ho To, Hin Fai Kwok, Kwok Kin Lai, Ching Po Lau, Chun Hay Ko, Ping Chung Leung, Kwok Pui Fung, Clara Bik San Laua. The in vivo and in vitro diabetic wound healing effects of a 2-herb formula and its mechanisms of action. Journal of Ethnopharmacology 2011; 134: 831–838.

Kirsner RS, Warriner R, Michela M, Stasik L, Freeman K. Advanced biological therapies for diabetic foot ulcers. Arch Dermatol. 2010; 146: 857–862.

Kit-Man Lau, Kwok-Kin Lai, Cheuk-Lun Liu, Jacqueline Chor-Wing Tam, Ming-Ho To, Hin-Fai Kwok, Ching-Po Lau, Chun-Hay Ko, Ping-Chung Leung, Kwok-Pui Fung, Simon Kar-Sing Poon, Clara Bik-San Lau. Synergistic interaction between Astragali Radix and Rehmanniae Radix in a Chinese herbal formula to promote diabetic wound healing. Journal of Ethnopharmacology 2012; 141:250– 256.

Larijani B, Heshmat R, Bahrami A, Delshad H, Ranjbar OG, Mohammad K, Heidarpour R, Mohajeri TMR, Kamali K, Farhadi M, Gharibdoust F, Madani SH. Effects of intravenous Semelil (ANGIPARSTM) on diabetic foot ulcers healing: A multicenter clinical trial. DARU 2008; 16(1): 35-40.

Leone S, Pascale R, Vitale M, Esposito S. Epidemiology of diabetic foot. Infez Med. 2012; 20: 8–13.

Morteza Nasiri, Sadigheh Fayazi, Simin Jahani, Leila Yazdanpanah, Mohammad Hossein Haghighizadeh. The effect of topical olive oil on the healing of foot ulcer in patients with type 2 diabetes: a double-blind randomized clinical trial study in IranJournal of Diabetes & Metabolic Disorders (2015) 14:38 DOI 10.1186/s40200-015-0167-9.

Moura LI, Dias AM, Carvalho E, De Sousa HC. Recent advances on the development of wound dressings for diabetic foot ulcer treatment: A review. Acta Biomater. 2013; 9: 7093–7114.

Nather A, Bee CS, Huak CY, Chew JL, Lin CB, Neo S, et al. Epidemiology of diabetic foot problems and predictive factors for limb loss. J Diabetes Complications. 2008; 22: 77–82.

O'Reilly D, Pasricha A, Campbell K, Burke N, Assasi N, Bowen JM. Hyperbaric oxygen therapy for diabetic ulcers: systematic review and meta-analysis. Int J Technol Assess Health Care. 2013; 29: 269–281.

Rice JB, Desai U, Cummings AK, Birnbaum HG, Skornicki M, Parsons NB. Burden of diabetic foot ulcers for medicare and private insurers. Diabetes Care. 2014; 37: 651–658.

Richard JL, Schuldiner S. Epidemiology of diabetic foot problems. Rev Med Interne. 2008; 29: 222–230.

Schaper NC, Apelqvist J, Bakker K. The international consensus and practical guidelines on the management and prevention of the diabetic foot. Curr Diab Rep. 2003; 3: 475–479.

Shahi SK, Kumar A, Kumar S, Singh SK, Gupta SK, Singh TB. Prevalence of Diabetic Foot Ulcer and Associated Risk Factors in Diabetic Patients From North India. JDFC. 2012; 3: 83–91.

Shufa Li, Jianyong Zhao, Jianping Liud, Fei Xiang, Debin Lu, Baoying Liu, Jing Xu, Huimin Zhang, Qian Zhang, Xianwen Li, Richeng Yu, Mingjun Chen, Xia Wang, Ye Wang, Bing Chen. Prospective randomized controlled study of a Chinese herbal medicine compound Tangzu Yuyang Ointment for chronic diabetic foot ulcers: A preliminary report. Journal of Ethnopharmacology 2011;133: 543–550.

Siersma V, Thorsen H, Holstein PE, Kars M, Apelqvist J, Jude EB, et al. Healthrelated quality of life predicts major amputation and death, but not healing, in people with diabetes presenting with foot ulcers: the Eurodiale study.Diabetes Care. 2014; 37: 694–700.

Snyder RJ, Hanft JR. Diabetic foot ulcers-effects on QOL, costs, and mortality and the role of standard wound care and advanced-care therapies. Ostomy Wound Manage. 2009; 55: 28–38.

Sumpio BE, Aruny J, Blume PA. The multidisciplinary approach to limb salvage. Acta Chir Belg. 2004; 104: 647–653.

Widgerow AD. Bioengineered skin substitute considerations in the diabetic foot ulcer. Ann Plast Surg. 2014; 73: 239–244.

Wraight PR, Lawrence SM, Campbell DA, Colman PG. Creation of a multidisciplinary, evidence based, clinical guideline for the assessment, investigation and management of acute diabetes related foot complications. Diabet Med. 2005; 22: 127–136.

Zhang J, Hu ZC, Chen D, Guo D, Zhu JY, Tang B. Effectiveness and safety of negative-pressure wound therapy for diabetic foot ulcers: a meta-analysis. Plast Reconstr Surg. 2014; 134: 141–151.